PRACTICAL

EAR-NEEDLING

THERAPY

MEDICINE & HEALTH PUBLISHING CO.

PRACTICAL

EAR-NEEDLING THERAPY

Published in Hong Kong by
Medicine & Health Publishing Co.
52 Tanner Road 1/F.
Printed in Hong Kong by
Ngai Shing Printing Co.
A4, 16/F., Fortune Factory Building
40 Lee Chung Street, Chai Wan

© December 1991   HK$80.00

實用耳針療法

ISBN 962-300-006-5

Introduction

THE DEVELOPMENT

OF AURICULOTHERAPY

Chinese traditional medicine considers that meridians (Chinglo) are passages ditributed in the human body, in which "blood" and "qi" (vital energy) circulate uninteruptedly, thus the auricle is linked up with every part of the body.

Meridians have the distributing features that externally, they connect with the body surface, by which the united relations among the auricle, four extremities and all bones are established, and internally, as the circulation of meridians is attached to the viscera, making the intimate interaction between the auricle and Five-Tsang (solid organs: the heart, lung, spleen, kidney and liver) and Six-Fu (hollow organs: the large intestine, small intestine, gall-bladder, stomach, urinary bladder and the three portions of the body cavity). Therefore, In a medical literature entitled "Wei Sheng Pao Chien" (The Health Treasure, published in the Yuan Dynasty, 1281 A.D.) stated: "Five-Tsang, Six-Fu and the Twelve Meridians all are connected with the auricle." This offers a marked explanation that the auricle and entire body are of a united whole cannot be separated. It provides the theoretical basis for following diagnoses and the treatment by means of the auricle.

The application of the auricle to diagnosis of diseases had been mentioned long ago in the earliest extant medical treatise in China. "Huangti, Nei Ching" (Canon of Medicine, compiled in the Warring States Period, 497-221 B.C.), of which the Chapter of "Lingshu-Shih Chuan" noted: "Inspect the auricle to diagnose kidneys"; also another medical literature entitled "Chong Chang Ching" (written in the Sung Dynasty, 960-1279 A.D.) mentioned the experience of judging prognosis by inspection of the auricle. Therefore we know that the diagnosis by the auricle has a history of about 2,000 years.

With regard to the record the treating diseases by the auricle it has been applied as early as the time of the early Warring States Period. In the Tsin Dynasty, a medical expert Ko Hung had quoted in his writtings entitled "Chou Hou Pei Chi Fang" (Prescription for Emergencies) that there was a physician called Chen Yueh-ren (in about 401-500 A.D.) who had treated a patient being at death's door by a method of blowing patient's left ear through a tube in three times, then so did to the right ear. In the same book, he mentioned also Chang Chong Ching's (in the late Han Dynasty) experience of curing a violent death with a method of pouring the juice of "xie" (Allium beteri) into the patient's ear. This indicates the fact that the application of the auriculotherapy has been recognized since very long ago. More records of the auriculotherapy can be found in "Chien Chin Fang" (written by Sun Szu-miao, in the early Tang Dynasty, 581-682 A.D.) stating "Insert or cautirize" the transverse pila above the auricular canal" (corresponding to the upper border of Ep Lower Abdomen) for the treatment of jaundice and epidemic viruses affected in the cold or hot seasons" and "Cauterze *Pt. Yangwei (Point

*Pt. stands for body point.

of the Eight Extraordinary Meridians) for curing tinnitus, etc.

In the Mid-Tang Dynasty, a medical literature "Chih Nieh Fang (written by Chen Chang-chi, in 730s A.D.) noted a prescription for relieving malaria by applying a piece of snake.s slough to fill both ears of the patient.

In the Yuan Dynasty, "Wei Sheng Pao Chien "stated: "Cauterize the small blue venule at the back of the ear for the treatment of infantile epilepsia".

In the Ming Dynasty, "Chen Chiu Ta Cheng" (Compendium of Acupuncture and Moxibustion, published in 1602 A.D.) had mentioned an experience of cauterizing the apex of the auricle to treat film in the eye.

Besides, in the rural areas of China, there had been spread many experiences about curing diseases by the auricle long ago. such as a method of kneading the auricular lobule for the treatment of red eye, pricking and causing bleeding on the veins at the back of the auricle with a needle for the treatment of swollen and painful eye, and stick to swear the helix a little with a pottery needle for curing costalgia and diarrhea. The moving auricular method of the massotherapy is with both hands to lift and pull the auricular lobule for the treatment of headache, and to knead the auricular lobule for curing infantile convulsion, etc. All the therapeutic methods noted above are effective. It can be seen that the application of the auriculotherapy has a long standing history.

Modern development of the therapy began in 1956 when the Laihsi County Hospital in Shantung Province obtained marked results in treating acute tonsillitis by the old folk practice of ear acupuncture. In 1957, at a seaside work-site in Amoy, Fukien Province, doctors effectively treated stye and some other eye diseases by pricking on the back of the auricle, causing slight bleeding. Based on studying the ear acupunture, making a conscientious observation on the relation between the auricle and every part of the body, applying it in the clinical practice, and supplementing more auricular points, P. Nogier, a French acupuncturist had developed the auriculotherapy.

Since 1958, the flowers of acupuncture treatment are in full bloom everywhere in China. The high tide of mass study and application of ear acupuncture had been arising, hundreds of clinical data have been summed-up, the range of the ear acupuncture has been extended and the contents of auricular points have been enriched. In a word, such a traditional treatmnet has been rapidly developed.

Up to now, the auricular points in common use has been increased to more than 200 in number. In a certain extent, the denomination and the practical application of points have reflected the contents of **the theory of Tsang-hsiang**[*] medicine and the antomico-physiology of modern medical science that provides rich experiences for the therapeutic method by combining Chinese traditional with Western medicine.

Of late years, further penetrating reaches on the diagnosis of diseases have been made, based on taking advantage of the reaction of auricular points, such as tenderness, congestion, changing colour of the skin, desquamation, papules, small blister, rottenness and increased reaction to conduction of electric current. And also the method of stimulating auricular points develops from simple insertion into the intradermal imbedding of needle, electrical-needle, drug iontophoresis in point, drug-injection, ear-point massage, kneading the ear

[*]The thoery of Tsang-hsiang

"Tsang" means the internal organs. "Hsiang" indicates the normal function of human body and the appearance of body surface reflected by pathological changes.

The theory of "Tsang-hsiang" consists of theory of Chinglo (Meridians) and theory of "Tsang fu" (internal organs).

with fingers, etc. The range of treatment has been continuously extended, the therapeutic effect has been increased, even the ear acupuncture anesthesia has been created. All of these have promoted the Chinese traditional medicine to enter a new phase.

CONTENTS

Chapter I

THE SUPERIORITY

OF AURICULOTHERAPY

Auriculotherapy has its superiority, such as quick effec-
tiveness, easy in manipulation, easy to learn and easy to
understand, economical and practical, convenient to patients,
less of side-effects and wide range of indication, etc.

In recent years, the therapy has been used in diagnosis,
differential diagnosis, prevention of diseases, and also used in
acupuncture anesthesia of surgical operation. All of thes have
obtained good results in varying extent.

(I) Wide Range of Indication

In their practice of starting out the ear acupuncture, the
Chinese medical workers have cured not only some functional diseases, but also some organic diseases as so-called
protracted "incurable" diseases. For Instance, functional
uterine hemorrhage, annexitis, aural vertigo (Meniere's
syndrome), neurodermatitis, cutaneous pruritus, anaphylactic
rhinitis, dysfunction of intestine, impotence, thromboangitis,
arteritis obliterans, disturbance of internal secretion, after-
effects of cerebral concussion, dwarfism, parotitis and otitis
medic, etc.

(II) Taking quick effect

Diseases respond to ear acupuncture the symptoms can generally be controlled in a short period, For Example:

1. To relieve pain quickly: Pains caused by wound (open-trauma), postoperation and inflammation like aprain, crushed injury, contusion, dislocation, fracture, ulcerated diseases, spasm of intestine, postnatal involution pain, urethral calculus, ascariasis in the biliary tract, generally, those diseases can be relieved within a few minutes.

2. To eliminate inflammation quickly: In the case of no suppuration, the developments of various inflammation can be controlled to reach the aim of eliminating inflammation within a few hours to 24 hours after the treatment, such as for the treatment of cholazion, hordeolum, furuncle, parotitis, pernio; bronchitis, pneumonia, tonsillitis, acute conjunctivitis, appendicitis, enteritis and dysentery, etc

3. To relieve itch quickly: Itching caused by dermal pruritus, anaphylactic dermatitis and prickly heat may be relieved and cured by auriculotherapy.

4. To give first-aid quickly: We have taken the view that the ear acupuncture is very effective in giving first-aid to patients suffering from shock, sunstroke or convulsion. Generally, the symptoms can be controlled and the blood pressure can be restored to be normal within several hours or even a dew minutes.

5. To reduce fever quickly: In the case of abiding high fever; the temperature can be restored to normal in half an hour after the treatment.

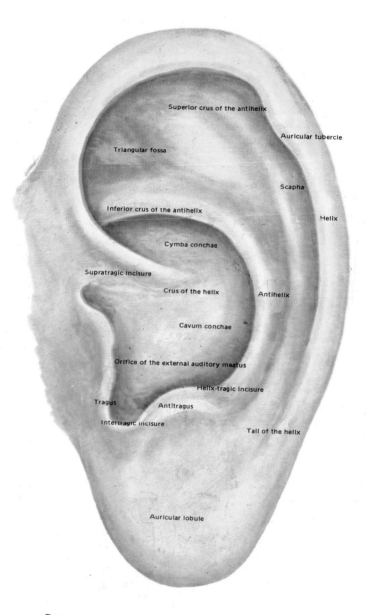

Diagram 1   Anatomical names of the auricular surface

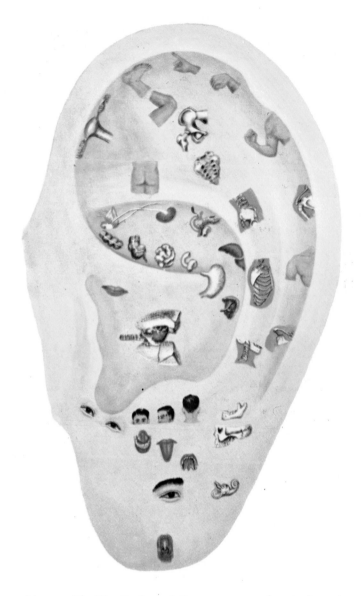

Diagram 2   Distribution of the appearance of auricular points

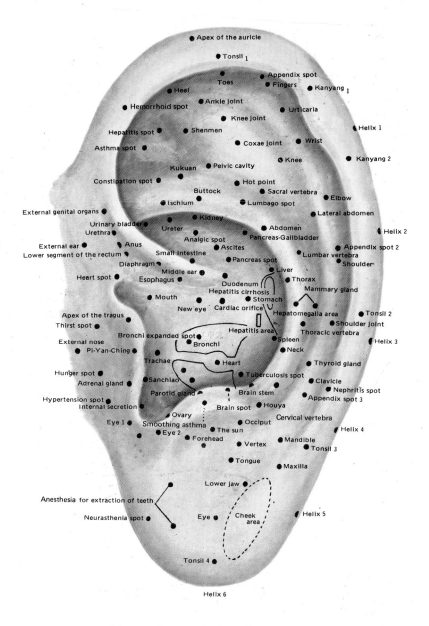

Diagram 3   Auricular points on the auricle

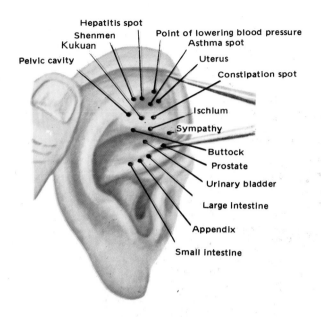

Hepatitis spot
Shenmen
Kukuan
Pelvic cavity
Point of lowering blood pressure
Asthma spot
Uterus
Constipation spot
Ischium
Sympathy
Buttock
Prostate
Urinary bladder
Large intestine
Appendix
Small intestine

Diagram 4   Auricular points on
the triangular fossa

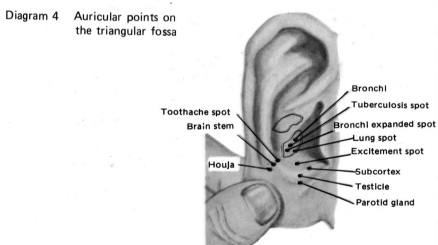

Bronchi
Tuberculosis spot
Toothache spot
Brain stem
Bronchi expanded spot
Lung spot
Excitement spot
Houja
Subcortex
Testicle
Parotid gland

Diagram 5   Acupuncture points on
the antitragus

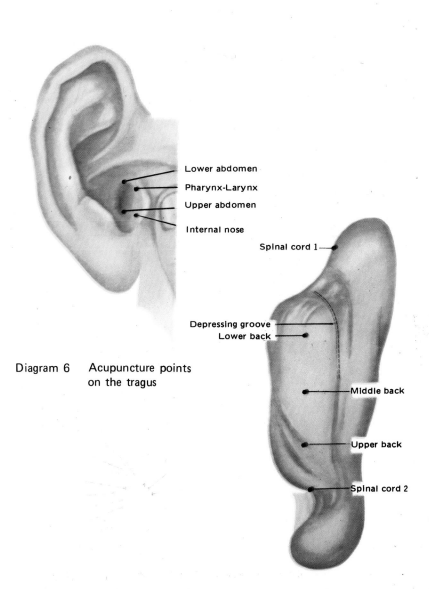

Lower abdomen

Pharynx-Larynx

Upper abdomen

Internal nose

Spinal cord 1

Depressing groove

Lower back

Diagram 6   Acupuncture points
on the tragus

Middle back

Upper back

Spinal cord 2

Diagram 7   Acupuncture points
on the back of the
auricle

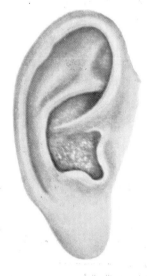

Desquamation of the lung area⟶dermal disease

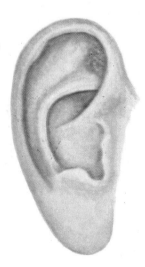

Papules or desquamation of the uterus area⟶gynecologic disease

Diagram 8　Inspection of the auricle

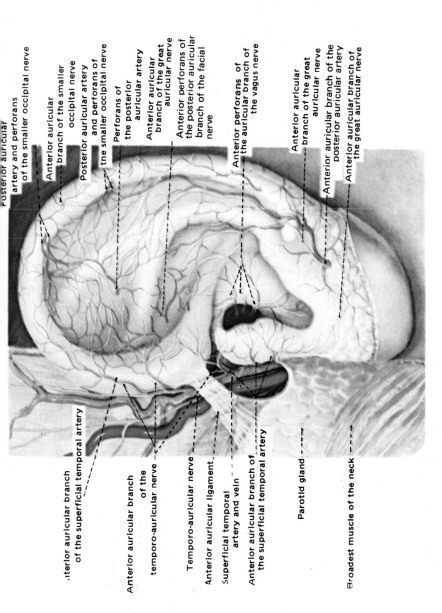

Posterior auricular artery and perforans of the smaller occipital nerve

Anterior auricular branch of the smaller occipital nerve

Posterior auricular artery and perforans of the smaller occipital nerve

Perforans of the posterior auricular artery

Anterior auricular branch of the great auricular nerve

Anterior perforans of the posterior auricular branch of the facial nerve

Anterior perforans of the auricular branch of the vagus nerve

Anterior auricular branch of the great auricular nerve

Anterior auricular branch of the posterior auricular artery

Anterior auricular branch of the great auricular nerve

Anterior auricular branch of the superficial temporal artery

Anterior auricular branch of the temporo-auricular nerve

Temporo-auricular nerve

Anterior auricular ligament

Superficial temporal artery and vein

Anterior auricular branch of the superficial temporal artery

Parotid gland

Broadest muscle of the neck

Diagram 9   The topographic anatomy on the anterior of the auricle

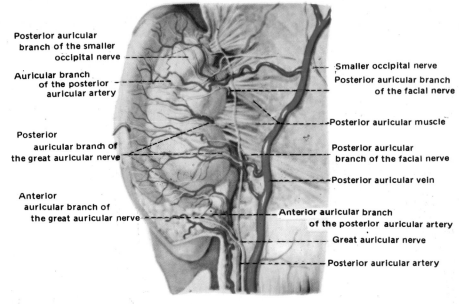

Posterior auricular branch of the smaller occipital nerve

Auricular branch of the posterior auricular artery

Posterior auricular branch of the great auricular nerve

Anterior auricular branch of the great auricular nerve

Smaller occipital nerve

Posterior auricular branch of the facial nerve

Posterior auricular muscle

Posterior auricular branch of the facial nerve

Posterior auricular vein

Anterior auricular branch of the posterior auricular artery

Great auricular nerve

Posterior auricular artery

Diagram 10 The topographic anatomy on the posterior of the auricle (superficial layer)

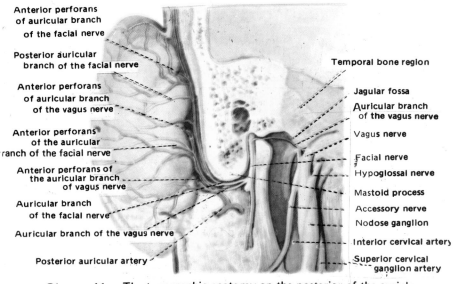

Anterior perforans of auricular branch of the facial nerve

Posterior auricular branch of the facial nerve

Anterior perforans of auricular branch of the vagus nerve

Anterior perforans of the auricular ranch of the facial nerve

Anterior perforans of the auricular branch of vagus nerve

Auricular branch of the facial nerve

Auricular branch of the vagus nerve

Posterior auricular artery

Temporal bone region

Jagular fossa

Auricular branch of the vagus nerve

Vagus nerve

Facial nerve

Hypoglossal nerve

Mastoid process

Accessory nerve

Nodose ganglion

Interior cervical artery

Superior cervical ganglion artery

Diagram 11 The topographic anatomy on the posterior of the auricle (deep layer)

(III) Simple in Manipulation

Ear acupuncture needs neither any equipment nor limitation of place and climatic condition, no matter where it is within doors, out of doors, workshop, construction site, battle field or class room, this treatment can be given. In the case if there is no acupuncture needle, a sewing needle may also be used instead of it. If necessary, the head of a match stick may be used to press with a force at the reaction point. This methods is also good for the treatment of headache, sprain, intercostal neuralgia and stomachalgia, etc.

(IV) Easy to Learn and Easy to Understand

Auriculotherapy is a kind of treatment by pricking needles into the auricle. The areas are concentric, the commonly used points are not so many and the distribution of auricular points have their definite order; many of the points are named after the anatomical names, easy to learn, easy to memory and easy to understand. Therefore, auriculotherapy has its own superiority. Persons who have only some medical knowledge will be able to master the technique within a short period. Hence ear acupuncture has relatively won the approval of broad masses, and is also easy to popularize and to push ahead. Not a few of people can grasp this technique to cure common diseases by studying in a short period. Some patients who had received auriculotherapy, their illness were not only cured, but also they themselves mastered the technique of ear acupunture, and they have given such a treatment to people around them with success.

(V) Economical and Convenient

Ear acupuncture requires only some needles and cotton ball with alcohol, but bring satisfactory results. People have praised the therapy for curing diseases without spending money and curing severe diseases with only a little money. Examination and treatment are much more convenient. In the process of the treatment, it does not interfere with study and work. If the patient can not be treated in time due to busyness of studying or work, he may be treated by using the method of intradermal imbedding of needle.

(VI) Less of Side-effect

In auriculotherapy, with the exception of some unusual pain during needling, there is not any specific side-effect. Sometimes, when the *Ep. Sympathy is inserted too deep, there is a feeling of heavy sensation in the location of Taiyang point. If Eps. Adrenal gland, Internal secretion, Heart, Kidney are to be inserted occationally there may appear some different symptoms, such as vertigo, fainting, palpitation, nausea, chilliness in lower limbs or numbness of general body; but when the needle is withdrawn a little, the symptoms noted above will then reduce or disappear in a little while. Phenomenom of needle-fainting only happens in few patients. If it occurs, let the patient lie down with supine position and he will be recovered in a moment. There may also be infection even atrophy of the auricle resulted from

*Ep. stands for auricular point.

unsufficient sterilization of the needles or the auricle. However, provided only that we work seriously, all these accidents can entirely be avoided.

(VII) Diagnosis and Differential Diagnosis

In recent years, great developments have been made on the diagnosis of auricular points, and some experience have also been obtained (for the concrete method, see Chapter VII and Chapter VIII). It is worth while to make reference to the differential diagnosis for acute abdomen of non-typical symptoms such as cyst of ovary, ureteral calculus, appendicitis and cholecystolithiasis, etc.

(VIII) Prevention of Diseases

Of late years, the Chinese medical workers have taken preventive treatment and obtained fairly good results for against parotitis, influenza and malaria. They took a comparative test on prevention of malaria by dividing the workers into two groups. They applied the ear acupuncture in the first group, begining from May, 1972, needling five auricular points: Adrenal gland, Internal secretion, Subcortex, Spleen and Liver, treated once every ten days, 12 treatments in all. The morbidity in this group was 1.2% in a year; while in the other group to which the preventive treatment was not given, the morbidity was as high as 8.5%.

We also found out : of the patients who had been treated under ear acupuncture80%had reflected that they had a good appetite, slept well and their resistance against illness was strengthening. Furthermore, they were seldom attacked by cold at ordinary times.

(IX) Used for Acupuncture Anesthesia

In recent years, the auriculotherapy has developed very rapidly. Patients are fully conscious during aperation when this kind of anesthetization is applied. Therefore, they can give play to their subjective dynamic role constantly strengthen and respond to the surgeons as the later require enabling speedy and successful operations, their confidence in overcoming the disease. In the case of patients who are in poor constitution, anesthetization by drugs are not advisable. while ear acupuncture anesthesia will ensures safe operations and the illness will be restored quickly.

At precent, ear acupuncture anesthesia is used successfully not only in removal of tonsils, extraction of teeth, but also used for operation of the thorax and abdomen, limbs, ears, nose, throat and eyes, etc. Hereafter, the range of indications will be more expansion.

In clinical practice, in addition to exertion of its active factors, we should also consider to combine it rationally with body-needling, Chinese medicinal herbs, Western medicine and other curing methods, when needed. By this way, the therapeutic effects of auriculotherapy will certainly be more excellent.

Chapter II

A BRIEF INTRODUCTION

TO THE APPEARANCE AND

THE STRUCTURE OF THE AURICLE

An auricle consists of the elastic cartilage of complicated form, a little of fat and the connective tissue covered with the skin. Under the skin there are distributed abundant nerves, blood vessels and lymphatic vessels.

The auricular concave faces forwords while its convex faces backwords. The base of the upper $\frac{3}{4} \sim \frac{4}{5}$ part of the auricle is elastic cartilage; and the lower $\frac{1}{4} \sim \frac{1}{5}$ part contents some fat and the connective tissue, it is called auricular lobute. The skin of the auricular concave adheres rather tight with the cartilage membrane.

(I) Anatomical Names on the Surface
of the Auricle (See diagram 1.)

1. **Helix:** The curved part at the most exterior circumference of the auricle.
2. **Crus of helix:** The transverse protrusion in the auricular cavity which is the initial part of helix.
3. **Auricular tubercle:** The protrusion of the postero—superior part of the helix.
4. **Antihelix:** At the inner side of helix, the protrusion

opposite to helix, the top of antihelix is divided into two branches.

5. **Superior crus of antihelix:** The superior branch of antihelix.
6. **Inferior crus of antihelix:** The inferior branch of antihelix.
7. **Triangular fossa:** The triangular fossa between the superior and the inferior cruses of antihelix.
8. **Scapha:** The groove between helix and antihelix.
9. **Tragus:** The lammellar shaped protrusion in front of the auricle.
10. **Supratragic incisure:** The depression between the superior border of the tragus and helix.
11. **Antitragus:** The protrusion of the inferior part of antihelix opposite to tragus.
12. **Intertragic incisure:** The depression between tragus and antitragus.
13. **Auricular lobule:** The skin lobe (without cartilage support) on the inferior part of the auricle.
14. **Cymba conchae:** Part of the auricular cavity above crus of helix.
15. **Cavum conchae:** Part of the auricular cavity below crus of helix.
16. **Orifice of the external auditory meatus:** Inside the cavum conchae.
17. **Interhelix incisure:** The depression between antihelix and tragus.
18. **Tail of helix:** On the border between the end of helix and auricular lobule.

(II) Nerve Supply on the Auricle

Nerve supply of the suricle is very abundant. The sources come from the trigeminal, facial, glossopharyngeal, vagus, great auricular and smaller occipital nerves, etc. (See Diagram 9–11), the distributed condition is as follows:

Anterior auricular branch of the temporo-auricular nerve: There are 3-4 small branches coming from the temporo-auricular nerve of the trigeminal nerve, spreading on the skin of the helix, anterior part of the triangular fossa, inferior crus of the antihelix, antero-superior part of the crus of the helix, cymba conchae, tragus and auricular lobule, etc.

Auricular branch of the vagus nerve: This starts from the jugular ganglion of the vagus nerve. After sending forth, it goes forwards to converge with the facial trunk within the facial neural canal. Having gone out from the mastoid foramen, the facial nerve leaves the facial trunk ascending along the posterior groove of the auricle; then it sends forth two perforans in the middle of the lower part of the groove, i.e. the anterior perforans of the vagus nerve perforate the auricular cartilage, dispersing at the cavum conchae and the external auricular canal.

Auricular branch of the facial nerve:
Having gone out from the mastoid foramen, it ascends within the posterior groove of the auricle and separates itself into the posterior auricular branch and the anterior perforans branch. The former distributes on the back of the auricle, while the later perforates the auricular cartilage and disperses in the cymba conchae, the postero-inferior part of the crus of helix and the middle part of the crus of antihelix.

The ending branch of facial nerve can also reach the lower part of the triangular fossa.

There are anastomotic branches in between the glossopharyngeal and vagus nerve. The auricular branch of the vagus nerve contents the fibres of the glossopharyngeal nerve, their distributed area may be the same as that of the vagus nerve.

The auricular branch of the vagus nerve goes a long distance within the facial trunk. Therefore, it can not exclude from the vagus nerve and the facial nerve having also the mixed fibres. There may be the vagus nerve and facial nerve distributed jointly in the cavum conchae and the cymba conchae. The exact distribution still await exploration.

Great auricular nerve:

This nerve sends forth from the cervical plexus, ascending along the surface of the sternocleidomastoid muscle in a height of the auricular lobule, then i nen it separates itself into the anterior auricular and posterior auricular branches. From which the anterior auricular branch perforates the auricular lobule to the anterior of the auricle (concave): The greater one ascends along the scapha distributed on the $\frac{2}{3}$ part of the scapha, antihelix, apex of the triangular fossa, cymba conchae and a part of the crus of the helix; the other one is distributed on the middle of the superior part of the scapha and the middle part of the helix. This nerve is also distributed on the skin of the auricular lobule where is the lower part of the intertragic incisure. The posterior auricular branch is distributed on the skin of the middle of the posterior part of the auricule.

The samller occipital nerve also comes from the cervical plexus, ascending along the posterior border of the sternocleidomastoid muscle, then sends forth some branches to the upper part of the auricle: The posterior auricular branch is distributed on the skin of the upper $\frac{1}{3}$ part of the posterior of the auricle. The anterior auricular branch and the perforans are distributed on the helix, the upper part of the scapha, the superior crus of the antihelix and a part of the triangular fossa. There is an anastomosis in between the great auricular and smaller occipital nerves, Therefore, the auricular skin is possibly ditributed by the fibers of the great auricular nerve passing through the smaller occipital nerve.

From the nerve supply on the auricle mentioned above we may perceive that the sourses of nerves in various auricular areas are not the same with each other, the helix, antihelix and scapha are mostly distributed by the great auricular nerve, only a small portion on the upper part of the auricle are distributed by the smaller occipital nerve. The nerves within the triangular fossa come from the auricular temporal, great auricular and smaller occipital nerve and form a neural plexus under the skin of the triangular fossa.

In additional to a few branches of the great auricular nerve, the nerves of the cymba conchae and cavum conchae are mainly distributed by the branches of facial, vagus and trigeminal nerves. These nerves are gathered here and form a neural plexus.

The nerve of the auricular lobute comes from the temporo-auricular and great auricular nerves. The smaller occipital nerve is distributed on the upper $\frac{1}{3}$ part of the posterior side of the auricle, and on the inferior $\frac{2}{3}$ part, is distributed by the great auricular nerve and the posterior auricular branch of the facial nerve. Besides, the auricular branch of the vagus nerve is also distributed on the posterior groove of Ep. Pressing groove of the auricle.

The auricular nerve in the derma forms a nerve net closely, which sends forth the nerve fibers to form the neurosensory endings in the epiderm, peripheral hair follicle and within the derma. In addition, the blood vessels are accompanied by a small neural bundle entering into the cartilage membrane and forming the neurosensory endings.

(III) Blood Vessels of the Auricle

The blood supply on the auricle is considerably abundant. It mainly comes from the superficial temporal artery of the external carotid artery and the posterior auricular artery. The superficial temporal artery sends out 3-4 anterior auricular branches nourishing the distributed areas of the anterior auricular branches of the temporo-auricular nerve. From the posterior auricular artery it sends forth the posterior and anterior auricular branches. Of which, the auricular branches are distributed on the posterior side of the auricle; paralelled with the facial, the posterior auricular branches of the great auricular nerve to nourish the posterior side of the auricle. The anterior auricular branches are paralleled with the anterior auricular branches of the great auricular nerve, then they perforate the auricular lobute to the anterior side of the auricle to nourish the distributed area of the great auricular nerve. (See Diagram 9—11).

The veins on the anterior side of the auricle are small, there are a great many of anterior auricular veins directly pouring into the superficial temporal veins. The veins on the posterior side of the auricle gather in 3-5 posterior auricular veins running from the brim to the root of the auricle, then follow into the posterior auricular veins.

(IV) The Lymphocinesis of The Auricle

The lymphatic vessels of the auricle are relatively abundant; most of them appear as a net in figure. The lymphatic vessels of the anterior side of the auricle flow into the lymphatic ganglion of the parotid, while most of the lymphatic vessels of the posterior side of the auricle flow into the lymphatic ganglion of the back of the auricle.

The content noted above may be offered some basic knowledge of the morphology for the exploration and study of the effects of the auricle in clinical diagnosis and treat ment. But we want to recognize the appearance and the structure of the auricle comprehensively, especially to make the course of meridians of the auricle clear that we have to carry on a great deal of science practice and take a futher study.

Chapter III

THE DISTRIBUTION

AND THE LOCALIZATION

OF AURICULAR POINTS

Auricular points are the location of positive reaction appearing on the auricle when the internal organs or the trunk of the body is affected by diseases. Needling such a location may obtain a result of treatment that is called "auricular points".

What the positive reaction points mentioned above are the particular locations on the auricle, manifesting a series resistance of reactions such as changing of colours, papules, deformities, desquamation tenderness and lowering of electrical etc. Therefore, they are also called reaction points, sensitive points, tender points or good conduction points, etc.

Treating diseases by ear acupuncture is noted down through the ages. Since 1956, the method has been used throughout China, and the points used has been increased to more than 200 in number (see Table 3—1 Diagram 2—7).

The distribution condition of the commonly used points on the auricle are briefly introduced as follows:

Table 3–1 DISTRIBUTION OF AURICULAR POINTS ON THE AURICLE

	Auricular-points	Anatomical regions	Explanation
Auricular Lobute	Lower Jaw	At the antero-superior part of the 2nd area.	Auricular lobute corresponds to the face region. Draw a level line from the brim of the cartilage of the intertragic incisure as a border line, then draw again downward two horizontal line, so the auricular lobute is divided into three equal parts. Divide again the highest level line into three equal parts, from there draw two vertical line, thus the auricular lobute becomes nine areas.
	Upper Jaw	At the postero-inferior part of the 2nd area.	
	Tongue Shang-He (Maxilla)	In the midpoint of the 2nd area. In the midpoint of the 3rd area.	
	Hsia-He (Mandible)	In the midpoint of the superior line of the 3rd area.	
	Eye	In the midpoint of the 5th area.	
	Internal ear	In the midpoint of the 6th area.	
	Tonsils	In the midpoint of the 8th area.	
	Cheeks	Lying around the border line between the 5th and the 6th areas.	
	Anethesia for extraction of teeth	there are two points invidually at the postero-inferior part of the 1st and 4th areas.	

	Auricular-points	Anatomical regions	Explanation
Antitragus	Parotid gland	At the midpoints of one third of the middle brim of the antitragus.	Antitragus corresponds to the head region.
	Soothing asthma	At the apex of the antitragus (may locate at the middle of the brim of the antitragus if the apex of the antitragus is not prominent).	
	Testicle	About 0.2 mm. inside the Ep. Parotid gland at the medial side of the antitragus.	
	Brain-spot	At the middle of one third of the superior brim of the antitragus.	
	Occiput	At the postero-superior part of the antitragus.	
	Forehead	At the antero-inferior part of the antitragus.	
	The sun	In the midpoint between the line connecting Eps, Occiput and Forehead.	
	Vertex Subcortex	About 0.15 mm. below Ep. Occiput. At the medial surface of the antitragus.	
	Excitement-spot	In the midpoint between Eps, Testicle and Lung.	

			Scapha corresponds to the upper limbs.
Scapha	Clavicle	At the scapha with the same level of Ep. Neck.	
	Fingers	At the scapha above the level of the auricular tubercle.	
	Shoulder Joint	At the scapha, lying between Eps. Shoulder and Clavicle.	
	Shoulder	At the scapha with the same level of the supertragic notch.	
	Elbow	At the scapha, lying between Eps. Wrist and Shoulder.	
	Wrist	At the scapha with the same level of the auricular tubercie.	
	Nephritis spot Appendix spot	At the infero-exterior part of Ep. Clavicle. There are three points in all, the first is slightly on the superior part of Ep. Fingers; the second, on the superior part of Ep. Shoulder; and the third, on the inferior part of Ep. Clavicle.	
	Articaria spot	Lying between Eps. Fingers and Wrist (slightly towards the medial side of the antihelix).	

Auricular points	Anatomical regions	Explanation
Cervical vertebra	At the projection of the begining of the antihelix.	Antihelix corresponds to the vertebra.
Sacral vertebra	At the projection of the begining of the superior and inferior crus of the antihelix, divides Eps. Cervical vertebra and Sacral vertebra into two equal parts.	
Thoracic vertebra	Above Ep. Cercial vertebra, within the 1st equal area.	
Lumbar vertebra	Above Ep. Cervical vertebra within the 2nd equal area. Besides, there is a similar distribution area of Ep. Sipinal vertebra in the medial border of the antihelix.	
Neck	At the notch between the border line of the antihelix and antitragus.	
Thorax	At the antihelix, level with the supertragic incisure.	
Abdomen	At the antihelix, level with the lower border of the inferior crus of the antihelix.	
Lateral abdomen	At the external surface of the antihelix, about level with Ep. Kidney.	
Hot spot	Between Eps. Coccygeal vertebra and Lumbago, about level with	

Antihelix

Thyroid gland	Ep. Buttock. At the superior part of Ep. Cervical vertebra near to the scapha.	
Mammary gland	At either sides of the upper part of Ep. Thoracic vertebra. These three points become an equilateral triangle.	
Appendix spot	At the lateral border of the antihelix, level with Ep. Kidney.	
Lumbago	At the lower projection of the antihelix, level with Ep. Sacral vertebra.	
Superior Crus of the Antihelix Toes	At the postero-superior part of the superior crus of the antihelix.	The superior crus of the antihelix corresponds to the lower limbs
Heel	At the antero-superior part of the superior crus of the antihelix.	
Ankle joint	At the inferior part between Eps. Toes and Heel, forming a triangle.	
Knee	At the begining of the crus of the antihelix and the extero-superior part of Ep. sacral vertebra.	
Coxae joint	In the midpoint between Eps. Sacral vertebra and Toes.	
Knee joint	In the midpoint between Eps. Coxae joint and Toes.	

	Auricular-points	Anatomical regions	Explanation
Inferior Crus of the Antihelix	Buttock	At the midpoint of the superior border of the antihelix (slightly towards the posterior side).	The inferior crus of the antihelix corresponds to the buttock region.
	Sympathy	At the border line between the brim of the inferior crus of the antihelix and curved brim of the anterior portion of the helix.	
	Ischium	At the midpoint of the superior border of the inferior crus of the antihelix (slightly towards the anterior side).	
Triangular Fossa	Uterus	At the midpoint of the anterior portion of the triangular fossa just behind the anterior portion of the helix.	
	Shenmen	At the bifurcation of the crura of the antihelix.	
	Pelvic cavity	At the inner surface of the bifurcation of the crura of the antihelix.	
	Point of lowering blood pressure	At the border line between the superior crus of the helix and the antihelix.	
	Asthma spot	About 0.2 mm. lateral to Ep. Uterus.	
	Kukuan	At the brim of the inferior crus of the antihelix, Become an equilateral triangle with Eps. Ischium and Buttock.	

Consitpation spot	Near by the middle section of the antihelix, at the intero-superior part of Ep. Ischium, forming a horizontal line.	
Hepatitis spot	About 0.2 mm. lateral to Ep. Uterus.	
Peripheral Crus of the Helix		The peripheral crus of the helix corresponds to the digestive tract.
Mouth	At the posterior wall of the orifice of the external auditory meatus.	
Stomach	At the upper portion of the cavum conchae and just below the disappearance of the crus of the helix.	
Esophagus	At the upper portion of the cavum conchae just below the crus of the helix.	
Cardiac orifice	At the upper portion of the cavum conchae and just below the crus of the helix, the point lies behind Ep. Esophagus.	
Duodenum	Lying in the above of the crus of the helix oppositing to Ep. Cardiac orifice.	
Small intestine	At the lower portion of the cymba conchae and above the crus of the helix. It lies at the point where slightly lateral to one-half of the crus of the helix.	
Large intestine	At the antero-inferior portion of the cymba conchae and just above the crus of the helix.	
Appendix	Just above the crus of the helix and lying between Eps. Large intestine and Small intestine.	

	Auricular-points	Anatomical regions	Explanation
Crus of the Helix	Diaphragm	Above the crus of the helix, forming a vertical line between Eps. Mouth and Esophagus.	Crus of the helix corresponds to the diaphragm.
	Middle ear	At the external part of Ep. Diaphragm, forming a vertical line between Eps. Esophagus and Cardiac orifice.	
Cymba Conchae	Urinary-bladder	At the antero-superior part of the cymba conchae, just below the inferior crus of the antihelix.	Cymba conchae corresponds to the abdominal region.
	Kidney	Lying on the upper part of the symba conchae at the superior portion of Ep. Small intestine.	
	Ureter	Between Eps. Urinary bladder and Kidney.	
	Prostate	At the medial side of Ep. Urinary bladder. below Ep. Sympathy.	
	Liver	At the postero-superior part of Ep. Stomach.	
	Pancreas-Gallbladder	Between Eps. Liver and Kidney	
	Pancreatitis-spot Ascites-spot	At the lower $\frac{2}{3}$ part of between Eps. Duodenum and Pancreas-Gallbladder. Lying among Eps. Kidney, Pancreas-Gallbladder and Small intestine.	

	Analgic spot		
		At the upper $\frac{1}{3}$ part between Eps. Kidney and Small intestine.	Cavum conchae corresponds to the thoracic region.
Cavum Conchae	Heart	Lying in the centre of the deepest depression of the cavum conchae,	
	Spleen	At the extero-inferior part of Ep. Stomach area.	
	Lung	Lying around the circumference of Ep. Heart.	
	Bronchi	In Ep. Lung area.	
	Tuberculosis spot	In the centre of Ep. Lung area.	
	Bronchi-expanded area	At the lateral $\frac{1}{3}$ part of Ep. Lung area.	
	Trachea	Lying between Ep. Heart and the external auditory meatus.	
	Hepatic cirrhosis	Forming a striation in the centre of Ep. Hepatomegalia area.	
	Hepatomegalia	In an area located at the lateral side between the upper and lower part of Ep. Stomach, and just below the disappearance of the crus of the helix.	
	Sanchiao (the three portions of the body cavity)	In the cavum conchae and lying among Eps. Internal nose, Lung and Internal secretion.	
	Hepatitis-area	Slightly below the middle between Eps. Stomach and Spleen.	
	New eye-spot	Among Eps. Esophagus, Cardiac orifice and Lung.	

Auricular-points	Anatomical regions	Explanation
Internal nose	At the inner surface of the tragus, slightly below Ep. Pharynx-Larynx.	The tragus corresponds to Eps. Nose and Pharynx region.
Pharynx-Larynx	At the inner surface of the tragus oppositing to the orifice of the external auditory meatus.	
Adrenal gland	At the lower projection of the tragus (at the lower brim of the projection if only one projection is found).	
Apex of tragus	The upper projection of the tragus (at the upper brim of the projection if only one projection is found).	
External nose	In the middle of the root of the tragus.	
Thirst spot	In the middle of the line connecting the apex of tragus and Ep. External nose.	
Hunger spot	In the middle of the line connecting Eps. Adrenal gland and External nose.	
Hypertension spot	In the middle of the line connecting Eps. Adrenal gland and Eye 1.	
Pi-yan-ching	In the middle between the apex of tragus and Ep. Adrenal gland, above the cartilaginous brim of the tragus.	

Tragus

Intertragic Incisure	Internal secretion Ovary	In the bottom part of the intertragic incisure Lying between Eps. Subcortex and Internal secretion
	Eye 1	At the antero-inferior part of the intertragic incisure.
	Eye 2	At the postero-inferior part of the intertragic incisure.
	Points for raising blood pressure	Between Eps. Eye 1 and Eye 2.
		Intertragus corresponds to Ep. Internal secretion.
Super-tragic Incisure	External ear	In the depression in front of the supratragic incisure.
	Heart spot	In the depression of the apex of tragus.
		Supratragic incisure corresponds to Ep. External ear.
Helixtragic Incisure	Brain stem	In the midpoint of the helix-tragic incisure.
	Hou-ja	Lying between Eps. Cervical vertebra and Occiput.
	Toothache spot	At the inner surface of Ep, Brain stem opposite to Ep. Hou-ja.
		Helix-tragic incisure corresponds to Ep. Brain stem.

	Auricular- points	Anatomical regions	Explanation
Helix	External genital organs	At the anterior part of the helix, with the same level of the inferior crus of the anthelix.	
	Urethra	At the anterior part of the helix, with the same level of Ep. Urinary bladder.	
	Lower segment of the rectum	At the anterior portion of the helix, with the same level of Ep. Large intestine.	
	Anus	In the middle between Eps. the Lower segment of the rectum and Urethra.	
	Apex of the auricule	At the upper part of the helix and facing towards the terminal portion of the inferior crus of the anthelix.	
	Hemorrhoid spot	At the medial side of the apex of the auricle, just above Ep. Point for lowering blood pressure.	
	Tonsils 1	Lying in the superior margin of the helix, vertically above Ep. Tonsils 4 on the auricular lobute.	
	Tonsils 2	At the helix, becomes an equilateral triangle with Eps. Tonsils 1 and Tonsils 4.	

Tonsils 3	Between Eps. Tonsils and Tonsils 2, on the auricular lobute.
Kanyang 1	At the helix, above the level of the auricular tubercle.
Kanyang 2	At the helix, on the lower margin of the auricular tubercle.
Helix 1, 2, 3, 4, 5, 6.	At equal intervals of six segments begining from the auricular tubercle of the helix downward to the middle of the lower margin of the auricular lobute.
Small occipital nerve	At 0.2 mm. of the medial surface of the upper margin of the auricular tubercle of the helix.
Upper back Middle back	At the upper cartilaginous eminence. Lying between Eps. Upper back and Lower back.
Lower back	At the lower cartilaginous eminence.
Depressing groove	A curved vertical groove on the back of the auricle.
Spinal cord 1	At the highest margin of the root of the auricle.
Spinal cord 2	In front of the mastoid process and at the lower margin of the root of the auricle.

Back of the Auricle

Auricular-points		Anatomical regions	Explanation
Others	Upper abdomen	At the inferior wall of the orifice of the external auditory meatus.	
	Lower abdomen	At the superior wall of the orifice of the external auditory meatus.	
	Point of support	In the midpoint of the vertical line between Eps. Urinary bladder. and Brain stem	

Chapter IV

THE FUNCTIONS OF

THE COMMONLY USED AURICULAR POINTS

"Often correct knowledge can be arrived at only after many repetitions of the process leading from matter to consciousness and then back to matter, that is, leading from practice to knowledge and the back to knowledge". This holds good in the investigation of the functions of auricular points.

In great deal of clinical practice we have realized that knowledge of the functions of auricular points should be acquired both by studying their personality and by studying their community. In the process of using these dual nature to estimate the functions of auricular points we feel never to arduous the position and the action of auricular points in treatment. The correct reconizing and correct handling of contradictory movement (internal relation) between them has great influence on the transformation of diseases. We hold that most of the points on the auricle not only have the intrinsic function endowed by the anatomical denomination of Western medicine, but also have abundant contents implied in the theory of Chinglo *(Meridians) and the theory of Tsang-hsiang depending on the theory of Chinese and modern medical science, we have both integrated the knowledge of the function of auricular points and their interrelation through a great deal of clinical practice.

The following is our preliminary knowledge of the fucntions of auricular points:

[Heart]

This point has the functions of "calming down the heart and the mind, regulating the blood and eliminating the heat of the heart". Main treatment: heart trouble, short of breath and chest pain. "The heart governs the energy and the blood" therefore it may be used in treating diseases of the cardio-vascular system. "The heart mantains the spirit, its function is related to the secretion of sweat", thus it is also effective in cases of high sweat, insomnia, dreams, amnesia, neurasthenia and mental diseases, etc. "The heart shows itself on the tongue", its meridian circulates and passes through either sides of the pharynx and larynx, hence it has also some significance in treating diseases of chronic pharyngitis, hoarseness, tongue pains, glossitis and stomatitis, etc.

[Liver]

The functions of the point are, "to promote the liver and the gall bladder, to drive out the evil wind to regulate the

* The theory of Chinglo :   Chinglo is the transport pathway of "Chihsueh — blood and chi (vital energy), in the human body, including the two large parts of "Chingmo" (Meridians) and "Lomo" (Conjunctive channels). The Meridian is a straight forward trunk, the conjunctive channel is the transverse branch. Chinglo in the inner part of the human body is related with the Five Tsang and the Six-fu; in the outer part is related with the five senses and the seven holes, the four limbs and the numerous bones, the skin, the hair, the tendon and the muscles. They cover up the whole body. "Chihsueh" is unimpededly in circulation along Chinglo so that every organic tissue in the human body is relating, coordinating with and regulating each other, the structure becomes a uniform whole. The chihsueh in Chinglo is poured out and distributed on localities of the body surface, these are called acupuncture points. The acupuncture points have the function of receiving stimulations. When needling the acupuncture points, Chinglo transfers these stimulations received by the acupuncture points and regulates the function of Chihsueh which excerts a curing result.

blood, to brighten the eyes and to help the stomach". Main treatment: acute and chronic hepatitis, cholecystitis, ictero-dermal pruritus. "The liver governs the muscles", however, it is applicable to diseases of hemiplegia, myasthenia and various sprains resulting from dizziness, convulsions, cerebro-vascular accident, etc. "The liver stores the blood", so that it is also indicated in treating blood diseases. hemorrhagic diseases and hypoferric anemia, etc. "The liver shows itself on the eyes", accordingly it has some properties in treating diseases of ophthomologic diseases. Furthermore, the meridian of the liver clasps the stomach, that is why it is effective in the case of the digestive system. "The liver con-trols the excretion", its meridian-energy retains under the armpit, therefore it can be used to treat fullness of chest, intestinal distention, painful menstruation and nolancholy emotions, etc.

[Spleen]
"The spleen governs the transportation and di-gestion, having the functions of digestion food, growing the boood, nourishing the muscles, strengthening the spleen and increasing the vitality". Main treatment: indigestion, gastritis and gastro-duodenal ulcers, etc. "The spleen commands the blood" so that it can be used in treating memorrhagic and blood diseases and anemia, etc. "The spleen governs the muscles as the vicissitudes of its functions always reflected on the mouth and the lips", hence it may be used in treating diseases of defervescent stage of muscular atrophy, stomatitis and stomatocace caused by underneurishment of the muscles, muscular pypotonic and various origins. Furthermore it is also effective in disorders of prolapse of anus, visceroptosis caused by the descending "central energy" and chronic diarrhea caused by the positive spleen in inadequacy, etc.

[Lung]

This point "governs the air and controles the respiration", having the functions of "pushing the circulation of the blood and the energy, facilitating the urination, nourishing the debility and eliminating the heat". Main treatment: diseases of the respiratory system, such as pulmonary tuberculosis, caugh, asthma, as well as edema caused by disturbances of general and lesser circulation. "The lung controles the whole body surface, converging its functions on the hair and the skin" so it is effective in diseases of common cold, night sweat, cold sweat and various kinds of dermal diseases. The meridian of the lung goes out of the throat, hence it can be used in treating hoarseness and pharyngolaryngitis.

"The lung and the large intestine are communicated with each other, forming the exterior—interior relationship" and the meridian of the lung descends to connect with the large intestine, that is why it is indicated in diseases of enteritis, dysentery, as well as those of stomatitis and stomatocace.

In ear-acupuncture anesthesia, this is a principal point to be used to increase the analgesia in the incising of skin.

[Kidney]

This point has the functions of strengthening the positive energy, helping the essense, promoting the lumbar vertebraew, conserving the cerebral cord. facilitating the "water ways" (the urethra), and increasing the sense of vision and hearing, etc. Main treatment: Nephritis, pyshonephritis, poor function of kidney, cystitis and diseases of the generative system (i.e. impotence, nocturnal pollution and gynecologic diseases), etc.

"The kidney shows itself on the ears and governs the bones; the essence of the bone is the pupils" so it can be used in treating deafness, tinnitus, impairing of hearing, diseases of the ophthalmology and relieving pain in fracture.

"The teeth are the remainder of the bone", "The kidney stores the essence, the essence produces the maroow" and "The brain is the sea of the marrow". Therefore, stimulation of this point has the therapeutic properties in treating diseases of looseness or bleeding of teeth and diseases of the mental and nervous system as well as those of neurasthenia and headache, etc.

"The kidney shows itself on the hair", thus it is also effective in disorders of alopecia and pelade.

Chinese traditional medicine takes the view that "The kidney is the congenital sourses", "The kidney and the urinary bladder are communicated with each other, forming the exterior-interior relationship" and "The kidney is the active basis of the human body". In addition the point is benificial to the digestion of food", thus it can be used in restoring lack of appetite as well as those of chronic and asthenic diseases. Meanwhile, "The kidney shows itself on two "Yin" (i.e. the organs of excretion— the genital organs and the anus), so it can be used to treat constipation.

[Large Intestine]

The main functions of the point are "to excrete the dregs carring downwards from the small intestine". Main treatment: dysentery, enteritis, diarrhea, appendicitis, constipation and incontinence of feces, etc.

The large intestine and the small intestine all belong to the stomach and the digestive system, hence it is effective in diseases of indigestion.

"The large intestine and the lung are communicated with each other, forming the exterior —interior relationship" and its meridian connects with the lung, accordingly, it can also be used in the case of the respiratory system.

[Small Intestine]

This point has the functions of "digesting all the ripe food and separating the nutriment and the dregs", its meridian reaches the stomach. Stimulation of this point has the properties of treating diseases of diarrhea, indigestion, poor absorption function of gastro-intestine, abdominal distention and intestinal tuberculosis, etc.

"The small intestine and the heart are communicated with each other, forming the exterior—interior relationship", and its meridian connects with the heart, therefore it can be used in treating diseases of heart troubles, such as palpitation, short of breath. "The meridian of the small intestine controls diseases which caused by the fluid" and due to its meridian circulates the neck, thus it has the properties in treating diseases of shortage of breast milk, sore pharyny and swollen neck.

[Stomach]

The functions of the point are "to receive and digest food", "The stomach and the spleen[are communicated with each other, forming the exterior—interior relationship". Main treatment: gastric ulcer, chronic gastritis, gastroneurosis, indegestion, lack of appetite and gastroxia or the reverse.

"The stomach has also a passage function". If the stomach is to be calmed. disorders of nausea and vomiting, etc. caused by the energy of stomach converting upwards will be restored.

The meridian of the stomach enters the teeth then follows the natural line of the hair and reaches the forehead and cranium. Therefore Ep. Stomach is also indicated in diseases of frontal headache and that of the nervous system like epilepsy, hysteria, schizophrenia, insomnia and toothache, etc.

[Gallbladder]

The functions of the point are "to reserve the bile". "The gallbladder and the liver are communicated with each other, forming the exterior—interior relationship", accordingly it is used in treating diseases of cholecystitis, ascariasis in the biliary tract, cholecystolithiasis and icterepatitis, etc. The meridian of the gallbladder runs over the neck to the temple and then reaches the front of the ears, hence it is also effective in diseases of deafness, tinnitus, dreams, migraine and rigidity of neck, etc.

[Urinary bladder]

The functions of the point are "to contain the fluid (urine)". "The urinary bladder and the kidney are communicated with each other, forming the exterior—interior relationship". It is usually used in treating diseases of acute and chronic cystitis, pyelonephritis, glomerular nephritis, prostatitis, enuresis, incontinence of urine, precipitant urination, frequent micturition and retention of urine, etc.

The neridian of the urinary bladder flows the posterior side of the thigh around the buttock then passes through the loins and the back reaching the head, finally enters the brain, accordingly it is used to treat haedache, lumbago, sore back sciatica, neurasthenia and insomnia, etc.

[Sanchiao]

This point brings together the effects of internal organs in the body cavity". Stimulation of this point has the properties in treating diseases of the circulatory and generative systems, heart and chest troubles, pain in flank and armpit, short of breath, indegestion, anemia, hepatitis, abdominal distention, dysfunction of abdorption and peritonitis, etc. Sanchiao has

Sanchiao has also another action in facilitating the "water ways" (urethra), for this reason it may be used in treating diseases of edema caused by various origins. The meridian of Sanchiao (Triple Warmer) circulates along the middle of the lateral side of the arms, thus it is also effective in relieving the pain in arms.

[Shenmen]

This point has the functions of "calming down the heart and the mind, and relieving pain". It is usually used in treating diseases of pain caused by insomnia, vexation, common schizophrenia, anaphylactic diseases and various origins. This is a principal point of relieving pain used in acupuncture anesthesia. Stimulation of this point has some properties in driving off the heat and counteracting poison, so that it is effective in treating inflammation. In addition, the point is has also another action against cough, hence it can be used to treat dry cough (but not suitable for moist cough), and bronchial asthma as well as those of epilepsy and hypertension.

[Sympathy]

This point is used in the treatment of some diseases caused by disturbances of the vegetable nerve. It has a strong action upon analgesia and spasmolysis of internal organs, such as griping pain caused by ulcers, ascariasis in the biliary tract, cholecystolithiasis and urethral calculus, etc. Being effective in relaxing the blood vessels, it is usually used in the treating diseases of pulseless disease, vasculitis, angina pectories caused by arterial and venous vasospasm or vasostenosis, and is also indicated in cases of arthmia, extrasystole, premature contraction, night sweat, cold sweat and eye diseases. Besides, in acupuncture anesthesia this is a principal point applied in thoracic and abdominal operation.

[Adrenal Gland]

This point is a representative area of the adrenal gland and adrenal cortex, having the functions of regulating the adrenal gland and cortical hormone. It is usually used in eliminating inflammation, decreasing swelling, anti allergy, anti rheumatism, anti infection and anti shock. Stimulation of this point has properties in regulating vasodilatation or vasoconstriction and stopping bleeding, so that it is usually used in treating diseases of hyperstension and pypotension, pulseless disease, vasculitis, and capillary hemorrhage or staxis, etc. and is also indicated in reducing high fever and low fever with indistinct origins. Furthermore, this point is also effective in stopping cough, soothing asthma and some dermal diseases.

[Internal Secretion]

This point is a representative area of the endocrine system. It is usually used to regulate various kinds of diseases caused by the endocrine disturbances, is also indicated in anti allergy and anti rheumatism.

Furthermore it is also used in treating some dermal diseases, and diseases of the urinary and gynecologic system, blood diseases, absorption disturbances of the gastrointestinal tract and malaria.

[Subcortex]

This is a representative area of the cerebral cortex, having an action of regulating the excitement or inhibition of the cerebral cortex. It is used in various syndrome caused by the irregulating excitement or inhibition of the cerebral cortex, and also effective in diseases of visceroptosis, as well as sedation, relieving pain, eliminating inflammation, decreasing swelling, stopping sweat and anti shock, etc.

[Occiput]
This point is usually used in treating diseases of the nervous system and meningeal irritation, such as convulsion, opisthotonos, trismus, rigidity of neack, neck pains, anti shock and for emergent rescue. Stimulation of this point has also the properties in preventing and treating train-sickness and seasickness, and is effective in cases of hyperopia and dermal diseases as well as for those eliminating inflammation, sedation, relieving pain, stopping cough and soothing asthma, etc.

[Brain stem]
This is a representative area of the medulla oblongata and the brain stem, having an action of spasmolysis and driving out the "wind". It is more effective in diseases of meningeal irritation such as opisthotonos, and is benefit to the brain and the mind—that is why it can be used in cases of atelencephalia and after-effects of cerebral concussion and after-effects resulting from cerebral meningitis as well as anti shock, anti allergy, relieving pain and stopping bleeding, etc.

[Brain spot]
This is a representative area of the pituiary gland. It is used in the treatment of various diseases caused by the dysfunction of the pituiary gland, such as dwarfism, hypertrophy in the ends of extremities, diabetes insipidus, hypermenorrhea, functional uterine hemorrhage, etc. and is also indicated in

cases of soothing asthma and hypnosis. Furthermore, it has also some properties in treating diseases of enuresis and vasculitis.

[Pancreatitis Spot]

Main treatment: pancreatitis, indigestion diabetes and mignaine.

[Uterus]

Main treatment: endometritis, velvitis, functional uterine hemorrhage, irregular menstruation, leukorrhagia, postnatal involuation, dysfunction of sexuality, orchitis, epididymitis as well as in the case of oxytocia.

[Forehead]

This point has the functions of sedation and relieving pain, accordingly it is used in the treatment of forehead pain, neurasthenia, insomnia, dreams, rhinitis, and sinusitis frontal, etc.

[The Sun]

Main treatment: migraine, sleepy sickness and nocturnal enuresis caused by sleepy sickness.

[Parotid Gland]

Main treatment: parotitis, obstruction of parotid duct and dermal diseases, etc.

[Soothing Asthma]

This point has the functions of adjusting the respiratory center, anti allergy and relieving itching, etc. Accordingly it is usually used in the treatment of dry caught, asthma, dyspnea, short of breath, fullness of chest, anaphylactic pruritus etc.

[Testicle]
Main treatment: dysfunction of sexuality, orchitis and epididymitis, etc.

[Ovary]
Main treatment: dysfunction of sexuality, irregular menstruation, overitis, salpingitis and sterility, etc.

[Excitement Spot]
Main treatment: sleepy sickness and anuresis caused by sleepy sickness, etc.

[Ascites Spot]
Main treatment: ascites and abdominal distention caused by hepatic cirrhosis and nephropathic syndromé, etc.

[Pharynx and Larynx]
Main treatment: chronic pharyngolaryngitis, hoarseness, pendulous palate edema, tonsillitis, aphasia, bronchitis and bronchial asthma, etc.

[Internal Nose]
Main treatment: various kinds of rhinitis, sinusitis, ulcerous vestibulum nasi, fruncle of nasal canal and common cold, etc.

[Diaphragm]
Main treatment: musculophrenic spasm, blood and dermal diseases. Besides, it has some properties in treating diseases of visceral hemorrhage and hemoptysis, etc.

[Middle Ear]
The same as Sanchiao.

[Apex of the Auricle]
This point is mainly used to let blood, once 2—3 drops of blood, It is effective in reducing fever, lowering blood pressure, eliminating inflammation, decreasing ammonemia, restoring hepatic coma. In addition, it has the properties in cases of sedation and relieving pain.

[Lower segement of the Rectum]
Main treatment: tenesmus caused by internal and external hemorrhoids, prolapse of anus, incontinence of feces and dysentery, etc.

[Urethra]
Main treatment: urethritis, urethrorrhea and urethrostenosis, etc.

[External Genital Organs]
Main treatment: inflammation of glans penis, eczema of scrotum, impotence and painful low lack and legs.

[Tonsil 1, 2, 3, 4]
Main treatment: tonsillitis and pharyngoLayngitis, etc.

[Hexlix 1, 2, 3, 4, 5, 6]
These points have the functions of eliminating inflammation, reducing fever, descreasing swelling and lowering blood pressure, etc. It is mainly used to let blood for the treatment

of tonsillitis and hypertension, etc.

[Kanyang 1, 2]
Main treatment: chronic hepatitis and also indicated in diseases of tardive hepatitis epidemic and S.G.P.T. that has not descended for a long time.

[Eye 1]
Main treatment: acute and chronic glaucoma, optic atrophy, etc.

[Eye 2]
Main treatment: various kinds of eye diseases.

[Eye]
Main treatment: various kinds of eye diseases, such as acute conjunctivitis, hordeolum, chalazion, keratitis, pterygium and ametropia, etc.

[New Eye]
Main treatment: ametropia and eye ground disorders, etc.

[External Ear]
Main treatment: deafness, tinnitus, hypoarcusis, and pernio and infection of the ear, etc.

[Internal Ear]
Main treatment: deafness, tinnitus, hypoarcusis, otitis media, furuncle of external auditory canal and Meniere's disease (aural vertigo), etc.

[Anesthesia for Extraction of Teeth]
This point is usually used in anesthesia for extraction of teeth and toothache caused by decayed teeth.

[Upper and Lower Jaw]
Main treatment: stomatitis, periodonitis and anesthesia for repair of cleft palate.

[Maxilla and Mandible]
Main treatment: toothache, anesthesia for extraction of teeth as well as those of mendibular arthritis and lymphadentitis of mandible, etc.

[Cheek Region]
Main treatment: trigeminal neuralgia, parotitis, facial nerve spasm, facial nerve paralysis, acne and furuncle on the cheek region, etc.

[Clavicle]
Main treatment: relieving pain for fixation of clavicular fracture, periarthritis of the shoulder and stenosis of cervical artery, etc.

[Shoulder Joint]
Main treatment: sprain in Shoulder joint and periarthritis of shoulder, etc.

[Shoulder]
The same as Shoulder Joint.

[Elbow]
Main treatment: sprain in joint, soreness of upper limb.

[Wrist]
Main treatment: sprain in wrist joint and gastric neuralggia

[Finger]
Main treatment: sprain in finger joint, finer inflammation and pernio, etc.

[Cervical Vertebra]
Main treatment: hyperosteogeny or involution of the cervical vertebra and prain in neck, etc.

[Thoracic Vertebra]
Main treatment: hyperosteogeny or involution of the thoracic vertebra, etc.

[Lumbo-Sacral Vertebra]
Main treatment: hyperosteogeny or involution of the lumbo-sacral vertebra and lumbo-sacral sprain, etc.

[Neck]
Main treatment: sprain in neck, hypothyroidism and hyperthyroidism and stenosis of Cervical artery, etc.

[Thorax]
Main treatment: diseases of thoracic cavity, intercostal neuralgia, chest pain and fullness of chest, etc.

[Abdomen]
Main treatment: diseases of abdominal cavity is also indicated in diseases of the digestive and gynecologic system, etc.

[Lateral Abdomen]
This point is commonly used for diagnosis. If Eps. Gall bladder or Kidney appear the positive reaction, there may have a feeling of tingling pain, it shows that the possibility of cholecystolithiasis or renal lithiasis is greater.

[Hot Spot]
This point has the functions of relieving pain and relaxing the vessels, especially it is indicated in diseases of acute lumbar sprain, pulseless disease and vasculitis, etc.

[Mammary Gland]
Main treatment: mastitis, shortage of breast milk and hypermastia, etc.

[Knee Joint]
Main treatment: rheumatismal arthritis o f knee, sprain in knee joint and relieving pain in patella fracture, etc.

[Toe]
Main treatment: sprain in toe joint, pernio and inflammation etc.

[Ischium]

Main treatment: sciatica, ischionitis, paralysis of lower limb and infantile paralysis, etc.

[Upper, Middle and Lower Back]
Main treatment: back pain and dermal diseases as well as relieving itching.

[Pressing Groove]
This point is mainly used in letting blood and lowering blood pressure.

[Spinal Cord]
Main treatment: amyotrophic lateral sclerosis and various kinds of paralysis.

[Smaller Occipital Nerve]
This point has the functions of sedation and relieving pain, is also indicated in diseases of spasm in cerebral blood vessels, after-effects of cerebral trauma, headache, vertigo as well as those of hemiplegia caused by hemorrhage and numbness of the hand caused by neurosis, etc.

Chapter V

AURICULAR POINTS USED IN COMMON DISEASES FOR REFERENCE

Table 5—1 Digestive System

Disease	Primary point	Auxiliary Point
*Nausea, Vomiting	Stomach, Shenmen, Occiput, Sympathy	Subcortex, Esophagus
Acute and chronic gastritis	Stomach, Sympathy, Shenmen, Spleen	Abdomen, Lung
*Gastro neurosis	Stomach, Liver, Sympathy, Shenmen	Duodenum, Smaller occipital nerve
Gastric ulcer	Stomach, Sympathy, Shenmen, Spleen, Lung	Subcortex, Duodenum
Duodenal ulcer	Duodenum, Sympathy, Shenmen	Stomach, Lung
*Gastric spasm	Stomach, Sympathy, Middle ear	Upper abdomen, Shenmen
Gastric ptosis	Stomach, Sympathy, Subcortex	Liver
Chronic cholecystitis	Gallbladder, Liver, Sympathy, Lung	Internal secretion
Chronic pancreatitis	Pancreas, Internal secretion, Sympathy, Shenmen, Pancreatitis spot	

Disease	Primary point	Auxiliary point
*Musculophrenic spasm	Diaphragm, Shenmen, Subcortex, Middle ear	
*Diarrhoea	Large intestine, Small intestine, Sympathy, Spleen	
Abdominal distension	Large intestine, Small intestine, Sympathy, Stomach	Abdomen, Sanchiao
*Enteritis	Large intestine, Sympathy, Small intestine, Lung	
Indigestion	Small intestine, Stomach, Pancreas-gallbladder, Spleen	Large intestine, Internal secretion.
Intestinal colic	Small intestine, Sympathy, Middle ear, Lower abdomen	
Gastro-intestinal dysfunction	Stomach, Large intestine, Small intestine Sympathy, Spleen	Sanchiao
Anaphylactic colitis	Large intestine, Internal secretion, Sympathy, Lung, Small intestine	
*Constipation	Large intestine, Lower segment of the rectum, Subcortex, Constipation spot	Sympathy, Spleen
Alcoholism	Occiput, Forehead, Subcortex, Smaller occipital nerve, Drunken spot	

Table 5–2 Respiratory System

Disease	Primary point	Auxiliary point
Cough	Pingchuan, Adrenal gland, Pharynx-larynx, Occiput, Lung	Shenmen
Fullness of chest	Sympathy, Heart, Thorax, Lung, Pingchuan	
*Chest pain	Points of the corresponding areas, Shenmen	
Common cold	Internal nose, Adrenal gland, Forehead, Lung.	
Bronchitis	Bronchi, Shenmen, Pingchuan, Adrenal gland	Sympathy, Occiput
Asthma	Sympathy, Shenmen, Pingchuan, Adrenal gland	Lung, Occiput
Whooping cough	Bronchi, Adrenal gland, Pingchuan, Sympathy	Occiput
Pneumonia	Lung, Thorax, Adrenal gland, Internal secretion	Subcortex
Broncho pneumonia	Bronchi, Sympathy, Pingchuan, Adrenal gland	Occiput, Internal secretion

Table 5—3 Circuratory System

Disease	Primary point	Auxiliary point
Hypertension	Depressing groove, Sympathy, Shenmen, Heart, let blood on the apex of the auricle	
Hypotension	Sympathy, Heart, Adrenal gland, Subcortex	
*Pulseless disease	Sympathy, Hot spot, Kidney, Heart, Adrenal gland, Liver, Corresponds to the locality, Subcortex	
Tachycardia	Heart, Sympathy, Shenmen, Small intestine, Subcortex	
Myocarditis	Heart, Sympathy, Shenmen, Small intestine, Spleen	
Hypoferric anemia	Liver, Spleen, Internal secretion, Diaphragm, stomach, small intestine	
Agranulosis	Liver, Spleen, Heart, Kidney, Internal secretion, Adrenal gland	Occiput, Diaphragm Sympathy
Premature contraction	Heart, Sympathy, Small intestine, Subcortex, Heart spot	
Coronary arteriosclerosis	Heart, Sympathy, Internal secretion, Adrenal gland	Small intestine, Kidney, Subcortex

Table 5—4 Nervous System

Disease	Primary point	Auxiliary point
*Headache, Dizziness	Occiput, Forehead, Shenmen, Subcortex, Smaller occipital nerve	
*Insomnia	Shenmen, Kidney, Occiput, Heart	
Dreams	Shenmen, Kidney, Occiput, Heart, Stomach	Sanchiao
*Migraine	The sun, Smaller occipital nerve, Shenmen, Kidney, Subcortex	
Trigeminal neuralgia	Cheek, Maxilla, Mandible, Shenmen, Occiput	External ear, Smaller occipital nerve
Facial nerve paralysis	Cheek, Smaller occipital nerve, Eye, Mouth, Subcortex	Liver, Occiput
*Intercostal neuralgia	Thorax, Occiput, Shenmen	

Disease	Primary point	Auxiliary point
Sciatica	Ischium, Shenmen, Kidney	
Ischiatitis	Ischium, Kidney, Shenmen, Occiput, Adrenal gland	
*After-effects of cerebral concussion	Kidney, Brain stem, Occiput, Shenmen, Forehead, Subcortex	Heart, Smaller occipital nerve
After-effects of cerebral meniningitis	Kidney, Brain stem, Occiput, Shenmen, Subcortex	Stomach, Heart, Smaller occipital nerve
Epilapsy	Shenmen, Occiput, Heart, Stomach, Subcortex	Smaller occipital nerve
*Neurasthenia	Kidney, Shenmen, Occiput, Heart, Stomach	Subcortex
Hysteria	Shenmen, Occiput, Heart, Stomach, Brain stem	Subcortex
Schizophrenia	Kidney, Shenmen, Occiput, Heart, Stomach	Brain stem, Subcortex, Smaller occipital nerve
Hysteric paralysis	Subcortex, Shenmen, Occiput, Heart, Points of the corresponding areas.	Stomach, Kidney, Smaller occipital nerve
Hysteric aphasia	Brain spot, Occiput, Heart, Shenmen, Kidney	Subcortex

Disease	Primary point	Auxiliary point
Facial spasm	Cheek, Shenmen, Subcortex, The sun, liver	Smaller occipital nerve
Shock	Adrenal gland, Occiput, Heart, Brain stem, Subcortex.	
Neural Hydro-dipsomania	Internal secretion, Sub-cortex, Shenmen, Kidney, Thirst spot, Brain spot	
After-effects of infantile paralysis	Points of the corresponding areas, Shenmen, Adrenal gland, Internal secretion	Subcortex, Occiput
Polyhirosis	Sympathy, Lung, Internal secretion, Occiput, Adrenal gland	
*Heat stroke	Occiput, Heart, Subcortex, Adrenal gland	Smaller occipital nerve

Table 5—5 Urinary and Generative System

Disease	Primary point	Auxiliary point
Precipitant urination	Bladder, Kidney, Shenmen, Urethra, Subcortex	
Pollakiuria	Bladder, Kidney, Shenmen, Urethra	
Retention of urine	Kidney, Urinary bladder, Sympathy, External genital organs	
Enuresis	Bladder, Point of support, Excitement spot, Kidney	Brain spot,
*Cystitis	Bladder, Kidney, Sympathy, Occiput, Adrenal gland	
Pyelonephritis	Kidney, Bladder, Sympathy, Liver, Internal secretion,	Spleen
Urethral calculus	Adrenal gland, Kidney, Sympathy, Subcortex, Urinary bladder, Ureter	
Acute nephritis	Kidney, Bladder, Sympathy, Liver, Internal secretion, Adrenal gland	Spleen

Disease	Primary point	Auxiliary point
Impotence	Uterus, External genital organs, Testicle, Internal secretion, Kidney	
Orchitis	Testicle, Internal secretion, Shenmen, Adrenal gland, uterus	External genital organs
Epididymitis	Testicle, Internal secretion, Shenmen, Adrenal gland, External genital organs	Kukuan, uterus
Premature ejaculation	Uterus, External genital organs, Testicle, Internal secretion, Shenmen	
Prostatitis	Prostate, Urinary bladder, Internal secretion, Adrenal gland, Pelvic cavity	
Diabetes insipidus	Urinary bladder, Urethra, Subcortex, Spleen, Liver	

Table 5—6 Endocrine System

Disease	Primary point	Auxiliary point
Hypophysial dwarfism	Kidney, Internal secretion Brain, Testicle (male). Ovary(female)	
Gynecomatism	Internal secretion, Brain, Mammary gland	
*Abscess of breast	Mammary gland, Internal secretion, Occiput, Adrenal gland	
Secretory disturbance	Internal secretion, Brain spot, Subcortex, Kidney, Testicle (male), Ovary (female)	

Table 5-7 Infectious Diseases

Disease	Primary point	Auxiliary point
*Parotitis	Parotid gland, Internal secretion, Cheek, Subcortex	
Varicella	Lung, Internal secretion, Adrenal gland, Occiput, Shenmen	
*Malaria (preventive therapy)	Subcortex, Internal secretion, Adrenal gland, Liver, Spleen	
Acute and Chronic hepatitis	Liver, Sympathy, Spleen, Hepatitis, Kanyang	Gallbladder, Internal secretion
Bacterial dysentery	Large intestine, Small intestine, Sympathy, Lung	

Table 5—8 Surgery

Disease	Primary point	Auxiliary point
*Neck pains	Cervical vertebra, Neck, Shenmen, External genital organs,	
*Periarthritis of the shoulder	Shoulder joint, Shoulder, Shenmen, Clavicle, Adrenal gland	
*Mammitis	Mammary gland, Internal secretion, Adrenal gland, Thorax	
Acute and chronic appendicitis	Appendix, Large intestine, Sympathy, Lung	
Ascariasis in the biliary tract	Gallbladder, Sympathy, Liver, Duodenum	
Anal fissure	Lower segment of the rectum, Lung, Large intestine, Spleen	
Internal and external hemorrhoids	Lower segment of the rectum, Large intestine, Subcortex, Spleen, Adrenal gland	
Prolapse of anus	Lower segment of the rectum, Large intestine, Subcortex, Spleen	

Disease	Primary point	Auxiliary point
Vaspulitis	Sympathy, Kidney, Heart, Adrenal gland, Liver, Spleen, Hot spot, Points of the corresponding areas.	Internal secretion
Pernio (1–2 degrees)	Points of the corresponding areas, Occiput, Spleen, Adrenal gland, Lung, Hot spot	
*Furuncle, Panaris, Carbuncle	Points of the corresponding areas, Shenmen, Occiput, Adrenal gland	
Erysipelas	Points of the corresponding areas, (*Tienchih), Occiput, Adrenal gland, Internal secretion, Lung	Shenmen
Relieving pain in fracture	Points of the corresponding areas, Shenmen, Kidney, Subcortex, Adrenal gland	
*Sprain, Crushed injury	Points of the corresponding areas, Shenmen, Subcortex	Hot spot
Habitual dislocation of joint	Points of the corresponding areas, Adrenal gland, Subcortex, Spleen, Liver	
*Acute cellulitis	Points of the corresponding areas, Adrenal gland, Shenmen Spleen	

Table 5—9 Gynemetrics

Disease	Primary point	Auxiliary point
*Dysmenorrhea	Uterus, Internal secretion, Sympathy, Kidney	
Leukorrhagia	Uterus, Internal secretion, Ovary	
Irregular menstruation	Uterus, Internal secretion, Ovary, kidney	
Amenorrhea	Uterus, Internal secretion, Ovary, Kidney, Liver	
*Parametritis	Ovary, Internal secretion, Shenmen, Uterus	
Endometritis	Uterus, Ovary, Internal secretion, Lung, External genital organs	
Chronic pelvioperitonitis	Uterus, Ovary, Internal secretion, Pelvic cavity	
*Postnatal involuation pain	Uterus, Sympathy, Shenmen Subcortex, Spleen	
Prolapse of uterus	Uterus, Subcortex, Sympathy, External genital organs	
Functional uterine hemorrhagia	Uterus, Brain spot, Liver, Spleen, Kidney Lung	Internal secretion,
Pruritus vulvae	External genital organs (Tienchih), Shenmen, Lung, Internal secretion, Occiput	Adrenal gland

Table 5—10 Otorhinolaryngology

Disease	Primary point	Auxiliary point
Trainsickness, Seasickness	Occiput, Stomach, Internal ear, Shenmen, Smaller occipital nerve	
*Furuncle of external auditory canal	Kidney, Internal ear, Internal secretion, External ear	
*Otitis media	Kidney, Internal ear, Internal secretion, Occiput, external ear	
Tinnitus aurium	Kidney, Internal ear, External ear, Occiput	
Hypoarcusis	Kidney, Occiput, Internal ear, External ear, Adrenal gland	
Epistaxis	Internal nose, Adrenal gland, Forehead, Lung	Press apex of the auricle
Ulcerous vestibulum nasi	Internal nose, Adrenal gland, Florehead, Lung	
*Simple rhinitis	Internal nose, Adrenal gland, Forehead, Lung	

Disease	Primary point	Auxiliary point
Anaphylactic rhinitis	Internal nose, Adrenal gland, Forehead, Internal secretion, Lung	
Hypertrophic rhinitis	Internal nose, Adrenal gland, Forehead, Lung	
Hoarseness	Pharynx-Larynx, Heart, Lung, Shenmen, Internal secretion	
*Uvular edema	Pharynx-Larynx, Shenmen, Adrenal gland, Lung	
Chronic pharyngitis	Pharynx-Larynx, Internal secretion, Lung, Adrenal gland	
Chronic laryngitis	Pharynx-Larynx, Heart, Internal secretion, Lung, Hou-ja	
*Acute tonsillitis	Tonsils, pharynx-Larynx, apex of the auricle, let blood on the apex of the auricle.	
*Pains after excision of the tonsilla	Tonsils, pharynx-Larynx, Shenmen	
*Meniere's disease (aural vertigo)	Kidney, Shenmen, Occiput, Internal ear, Subcortex	Stomach, Smaller occipital nerve

Table 5—11 Stomatology

Disease	Primary point	Auxiliary point
Barred teeth	Maxilla, Mandible, Tooth-ache, Kidney, Hou-ja	
Stomatocace	Mouth, Internal secretion, Shenmen, tongue, Lung	
*Toothache	Maxilla, Mandible, Shenmen, Toothache, Hou-ja	
Looseness of ~~tooth~~ tooth	Kidney, Maxilla, Mandible, Occiput	
Periodonitis	Maxilla, Mandible, Mouth, Adrenal gland, Kidney	
Glossitis	Tongue, Mouth, Internal secretion, Heart, Lung	

Table 5—12 Ophthalmology

Disease	Primary point	Auxiliary point
Hordeolum	Eye, Liver, Spleen	
*Chalazion	Eye, Liver, Spleen	
*Acute conjunctivitis	Eye, Liver, Lung	
Bollicular conjunctivitis	Eye, Liver, Adrenal gland, Lung	
Electric ophthalmitis	Kidney, Liver, Eye Shenmen	
Night blindness	Liver, Eye 2, Eye, Occiput	
Diffused light	Kidney, Liver, Eye, Eye 2, Occiput	
Myopia	Kidney, Liver, Eye 2, Eye, New eye	
Diplopia	Kidney, Liver, Eye 2, Eye	
Chronic glaucoma	Kidney, Liver, Eye 1, Eye 2, Eye	

Table 5–13 Dermatology

Disease	Primary point	Auxiliary point
*Folliculitis	Points of the corresponding areas (Tienchih), Lung, Occiput, Internal secretion, Adrenal gland	
Zona	Points of the corresponding areas (Tienchih), Lung, Occiput, Internal secretion, Adrenal gland	
Cutaneous pruritus	Shenmen, Lung, Occiput, Internal secretion, Adrenal gland, Parotid gland	
*Urtocaria	Shenmen, Lung, Occiput, Internal secretion, Adrenal gland	
Verruca vulgaris	Lung, Internal secretion, Occiput, Adrenal gland, Points of the corresponding areas (Tienchih).	
Neurodermatitis	Points of the corresponding areas (Tienchih), Lung, Occiput, Adrenal gland, Parotid gland	

Disease	Primary point	Auxiliary point
Dermatitis solaris	Shenmen, Lung, Internal secretion, Adrenal gland	
Anaphylactic dermatitis	Lung, Internal secretion, Occiput, Adrenal gland, Points of the corresponding areas (Tienchih)	
Miliaria	Lung, Adrenal gland, Occiput, Shenmen	
Alopecia areata	Points of the corresponding areas (Tienchih), Kidney, Lung, Internal secretion	
Alopecia	Kidney, Lung, Internal secretion, Occiput	
Dermatitis seborrhoica	Lung, Internal secretion, Spleen, Occiput, Adrenal gland, Kidney	
Rosacea	External nose (Tienchih), Lung, Internal secretion, Adrenal gland	
Acne	Lung, Internal secretion, Testicle, Cheek (Tienchih)	
Vitiligo	Lung, Internal secretion, Occiput, Adrenal gland, Points of the corresponding areas (Tienchih)	

Disease	Primary point	Auxiliary point
Verruca vulgaris	Lung, Adrenal gland, Occiput, Large intestine, Points of the corresponding areas	
Eczema	Lung, Adrenal gland, Occiput, Large intestine, Points of the corresponding areas	
Eczema in children	Points of the corresponding areas (Tienchih), Lung, Occiput, Adrenal gland	
Scleroderma	Lung, Occiput, Internal secretion, Adrenal gland, Liver, Spleen, Brain spot	
Mycotic stomatits	Mouth, Internal secretion, Adrenal gland, Occiput, Lung	

* The point has marked effects with a successful rate of over 90 percent.

**"Tienchih" (blood letting) with needle

Aiming at the point required, inserted the short needle Nos. 26—28 (or an ordinary hypodermic needle, prismatic needle or body scarificator) quickly about 1 fen deep, sway the needle to and fro several times and then withdraw the needle and let bleeding— this is called "Tienchih". This method is used for treating heatstroke, syncope, sore throat.

Chapter VI

THE MANIPULATION METHODS

OF AURICULOTHERAPY

The manipulation methods and procedure of ear acupuncture are generally as follows:

1. Detection of tender points

The therapeutic effect of ear acupuncture depends closely upon whether the tender points are accurately detected or not, and this is a key to success in auriculotherapy. Therefore when a patient is to be detected, we must diagnose him thoroughly at first, then detect the tender points according to the reaction areas.

When the test probe (a match stick can be used if a test probe is unavailable) is being pressed down on the point, the patient will have some reaction such as a frown of eyebrow, a wink of the eye, a cry of pain an avading movement, etc. While detecting of points the hand manoeuvre should be applied uniformly, slowly and softly in order to find out the exact reaction points. If in rare cases when we fail to find out the tender points, we may massage that area with fingers; then detect there again or detect the reaction area on the opposite auricle. If there is no reaction of tender points, we may then take a rest for a moment. And if there is still no result after detecting repeatedly, treatment may be taken with the method of selection of points according to the symptoms.

2. The amount of points and the course of treatment

Generally, once 3-5 points. Both auricles may be inserted at a time or the affected auricle only. The course of treatment is determined according to the condition of disease. Generally, 10 treatments to a course. After an intervals of 5-7 days, then go on with the second course.

3. Prior to treatment

The auricle should be wipe with 75% alcohol of cotton ball, from the interior side outwards, from superior portion downwards and from the anterior side backwards thoroughly to avoid infection of the auricle. A strict disinfection before treatment is required. If there is found inflammation at the inserted site after treatment, it should be wiped with 2.5% tincture of iodine. Puncture Eps. External ear, Adrenal gland, Occiput and Kidney, etc. if necessary. By doing so the aim of eliminating inflammation will be obtained.

4. While giving the treatment

With the left thumb, fix the periphery of the auricular point where the needle is to be inserted; while the posterior side of the point is supported with the index finger of the same hand in order to the depth of the insertion can be well controlled, the sense of pain caused by needling can also be reduced.

Advance the needle with the hand manoeuvre at a 180 degrees clock-wise, the procedure should be accurately and swiftly.

5. After insertion of the needle.

Generally, retain the needle in the position for 20-30 minutes or so, 1-2 hours or prolong a little in chronic diseases. In the process of retaining the needle for curing sprain in joints, rotate the needle 1-2 times for strengthening the stimulation. At the same time, let the patient move his joints of the affected side for increasing the therapeutic effects.

6. Withdrawal of the needle

If the inserted site appears bleeding, it should be stopped with a cotton ball. In clinical practice, it is often seen that Eps. Shenmen, Occiput, Internal secretion and Kidney are apt to bleed and so in the patients with hypertension and thrombopenia. During needling, attention should be paid in keeping away from those small blood vessels, but sometimes coming out of a few drops of blood do promote the therapeutic effects.

7. Practice proved

Applying a fine needle (hao-chen) Nos. 28 will get better results than that of Nos. 30. Sometimes good results can be obtained by using the method of one point inserted with several needles. In curing chronic disease and the diseases having been treated previously by various kinds of methods, the therapeutic effect is insufficient, the primary points may be inserted with more needles,. By doing so, a better result will be obtained.

Contraindications and Management of Needle-Fainting

Most patients accommodate to ear acupuncture and only rare patients may possibly have some varying extents of fainting during needling, such as vertigo, paleness, cold sweating and lowering of blood pressure, etc.

(I) Contraindications

1. A pregnant woman with habitual miscarriage, should not be treated with auriculotherapy, and for 5-9 months of pregnancy it is not suitable to adopt Eps. Uterus, Ovary, Internal secretion, Abdomen and Pelvic cavity to avoid causing of abortion or premature labor.

2. Patients, under the circumstance of over fatigus, hunger, extremely weakened physical condition or severe anemia, are prohibited to be treated with this therapy. If necessary place the patient in a recumbent position to avoid needle-fainting.

For an older patient with hypertension or arterosclerosis, when needling or puncture Ep. Depressing groove to let blood, in addition to let the patient has a bed rest for half an hour before the treatment, let him take a recumbent position during treatment. After treatment, the patient must be carefully observed for half an hour before he goes away in order not to cause any accident.

3. Pernio or inflammation of the auricle, on which needling is prohibited to prevent diffusion of inflammation. Keep away from the periphery of inflammation, when needed. Or insert Eps. External ear, Adrenal gland, Occiput and Kidney at first until pernio or inflammation having been cured then continue the treatment of the disease concerned.

(II) Management of Needle-fainting

The outstanding feature of needle-fainting is mainly manistested in fainting, paleness, cold sweating, lowering of blood pressure, etc. Methods of management are as follows:

1. In mild cases, it is not necessary to withdraw the needles out, let the patient has a rest for a while and offer him some warm drinks. At the same time console him so as to calm down his excitement.

2. In severe cases, the needles should be withdrawn immediately, place the patient in a lower head position, then insert the withdrawn needle into Eps. Adrenal gland, Subcorted, Heart and Occiput at once, after that the needle-fainting can be recovered by itself.

3. After needling, if specific pain of the helix, or other symptoms occur like headache, vertigo, panicky, vomiting, trismus, chill of lower extremities or numbness of whole body, which are mostly caused by inserting to deep in Eps. Adrenal gland, Sympathy or Internal secretion. Generally, after withdraw the needle upwards a little, what the symptoms above noted will be decreased or disappeared. But it the symptoms do not reduced, the needles should be withdrawn entirely, the symptoms will be diappeared.

Some Auxiliary Manipulation Methods

The following auxiliary manipulation methods are effective for treatment:

(I) Imbedding Needles in Auricular Points

There are two kinds of needles, i.e. the intradermal needle and press-needle. The needles are to be inserted and imbedded in the effective auricular points so as to produce the stimulation action without interruption. It is suitable for curing chronic diseases or patients who can not be received treatment every day.

[Methods]
1. Routine disinfection of the auricle.
2. Clip a intradermal needle or a press-needle with a forceps and insert it into the auricular point, while the tail of the needle or the needle-ring remaining upon the skin is fixed with a piece of plaster.
3. Imbed the needle once for 1-7 days.

[Precautions]
1. Ask the patient to press on the place where the needle is imbedded with his own fingers, 2-3 times daily for increasing the stimulation and strengthening the therapeutic effects.
2. In the hot season, this method is not to be adopted to avoid causing infection of the auricle.
3. In the duration of imbedding of needle, bathing or washing the head should be paid much attention never to soak the auricle.
4. 2-3 days after the imbedding of needle, if the auricle has a swelling pain which shows that there is infection on the auricle. To this, active measures should be taken:

(a) Selection of auricular points: External ear, Adrenal gland, Occiput and Kidney.

(b) Sulfadizine (S D), orally or injection with penicilin, the dosage of drugs given is as directed by the doctor.

(Please refer to Appendix 3)

(II) Injection of Drugs into Auricular Points

Injection of drugs into auricular points is a kind of treatment combining Chinese traditional and modern medicine by application of needling and drug therapy. Certain solutions without stimulant result used for injecting into the concerning auricular points and so making use of both by needling and drug solution to achieve a curing result.

The commonly used drugs: 0.5-1.0% of Dibucaine (Nupercaine); Vitamin B 1(Thiamine hydrochloride);Vitamin B 12; Placental tissue serum; Placental globutin; Heparin; Serum; Penicilin and Streptomycin, etc.

[Methods]

1. Routine disinfection of the auricle.

2. Selection of points and injection drugs depending upon the symptom.

3. Each point about 0.2-0.4 cc to be injected in between the cartilage and intraderma, a small pimple will appear on the area where injected.

4. Once every 2-3 days until a course consisting of 5-7 injections are given.

[Precautions]

1. Aseptic technique should be paid to avoid infection.

2. Stimulant drugs are seriously prohibited to avoid necrosis of tissue.

(III) Auricular Points Incised Therapy

This is a strong stimulant therapy, suitable for chronic and intractable diseases.

[Methods]

1. Routine disinfection of the auricule.

2. Advance the tip of a scalpel into the incision of selected auricular points about 0.2 cm. and let out some drops of blood, then wrap the incision with aseptic dressing. Once 2-4 points.

3. Treat once every 7-10 days, 3 treatments to a course.

[Precautions]
1. Be absolute of aseptic technique.
2. Within 3-5 days after treatment, bathing or washing the head are strictly prohibited to avoid infection of the incision.
3. Too wide and too deep incision are not allowed. If there is ineffective after 3 treatments, other methods of therapy should be replaced.

(IV) Auricular Points Picked Therapy

This is a strong stimulant therapy of auricular points, suitable for chronic and intractable diseases.
[Methods]
1. Routine disinfection of the auricle.
2. A sterilized presmatic needle is punctured into the subcutaneous cartilage of the auricle, then pick it up with a force. Once 2-4 points.
3. Wrap the picked points with some aseptic dressing.
4. Treat once every 3-5 days. 3 treatments to a course.

[Precautions]
1. The angle of the presmatic needle should not be too sharp, tearing the skin is considered to be against the rule.
2. In the duration of the treatment, bathing or washing the head are absolutely prohibited to avoid infection.

(V) Electric Stimulation Method of Auricular points

Making use of an ordinary medical electro-therapeutic apparatus and the inserted needles are linked with the source of electricity to stimulate auricular-points continuously to achieve the therapeutic effects. It is suitable for curing some chronic diseases and for patients who have not obtained a satisfactory result after receiving common acupuncture treatment.

[Methods]

1. When both ears are needled at the same time, the positive as well as the negative electrodes should firmly be held on each side of the needle-handle, supplying electricity for 10-15 minutes. The power output is considered appropriate when the patient gets a marked feeling of slight burning pain in the auricle concerned. If only one ear is inserted, one of the electrode is held by the patient's hand, and the other electrodes are all clipped on the needle-handle. The power output is the same as mentioned above.

2. When no needle is available, the test brobe may be used instead to press the auricularpoint, another electrode is held in the patient's hand. The power output is as mentioned above, supplying electricity for 2-3 minutes. Treat once every other day, 7-10 treatments to a course.

(VI) Massotherapy of Auricular Points

This is a kind of therapy by giving a massage to or pressing the reactive points on the auricle. The concrete procedure is as follows:

1. A method of pressing with a test probe

Make use of a test probe giving a slight pressure or massage on the reaction points of the auricle, 2-3 minutes for each point.

2. A method of pressing with the rape-seed

Put the rape-seed on he reaction points of the auricle, then fix it with a piece of plaster

3. A method of pressing with match-stick

Put a match-stick about 0.1-0.2 c.m. long, then fix it with a piece of plaster.

Introduce the second and the third methods to the patient and ask him to press the local by himself at least 3 times a day and take away the rape-seed after seven days.

Chapter VII

A BRIEF INTRODUCTION TO

INSPECTION ON THE AURICLE

Through a great deal of clinical observation we discover the fact that when certain internal organs or local area of human body suffered from illness, especially organic disease, the positive reactions will appear on the corresponding regions or definite areas of the majority of the victims . This pathological changes are symbolized by changing in colour of the skin, deformation, desquamation and papules, etc.

As of quite a few cases with gastric ulcer there appear a kind of pathological reaction, a small round spot within Ep. Stomach area of the auricle, by which it is obviously dinstinguished from the circumference of the normal skin: yet more of not a few patients whose stomach had been gasactomy , there can also appear a dark-red or white thread-like crescent scar on the auricular point concerned.

By analysing and studying earnestly a great deal of clinical practice, Chinese medical workers initially recognize the phenomenon of general pathological reactions of some diseases on the auricle, such as gastric disease, lung disease, acute and chronic appendicitis, hepatitis, tumor, gynecology and some skin disorders, etc. they give some terms of reference concerning assistant diagnosis and differential diagnosis of diseases.

Inspection on the auricle is suitable for the mountainous districts, rural areas and some medical units where are lack of medical equipments. It has a certain practical significance for promoting and preventing the health of masses.

(I) Method of Inspection

1. During inspection, following the anatomical regions of the auricle pull up the ear lightly with the thumb and the index finger to inspect it from above downwards, from outside inwards step by step.
2. When the positive reaction is found, support the back of the auricle with the index finger so as to bring the skin to the stretch and look at the positive reaction clearly.
3. In inspecting the patient's both ears, when it is found that the positive reactions differ from each other, they should be compared and contrasted with each other; directed against the regions, quality and the extent of pathological reactions, a dialectical and comprehensive analysis should be carried out to make a tentative diagnosis.

4. If the protuberence or nodules-like reactions are found, the physician may use his own hand or a test probe to detect the size and the hardness of the nodules and see whether they remove or not, whether their borders are in good order and tenderness or not, etc.
5. In inspecting the triangular fossa and the calvum conchae, use a test probe (or a match stick) to extend the crus of helix and expose the local region.

(II) The Reactive-Expression on the Auricle

Table 7-1 Auricular Reaction and Classification of Diseases

Reaction	Expression	Common disease
Changing in colour	(a) White spots or white fufurs with dark-gray or redish border. (b) White small spots with redish border.	Acute and chronic gastritis, gastric and duodenal ulcer, acute and chronic trachitis, liver and gallbladder diseases, nephritis, various kinds of arthritis, headache and vertigo, acute appendicitis, eye diseases, gynecologic disease, changing of blood pressure and cardiopathy, etc.
Deformation	(a) Depressed spots (b) Protuberant stripes or nodules.	Tubeculosis, chronic appendicitis, hepatomegalia, tumor, cardiopathy, osteanaphysis, traumatic paraplegia and transformation, hypertrophy or degeneration of vertebrae, etc.
Papules	white or red dotted papules (similar to the groose pimple)	Gynecologic disease, small and large intestinal disease, nephritis, cystitis, cardiopaphy, pulmonary tuberculosis, acute and chronic trachitis, etc.

| Desquamation | White furfurs showing rice-bran-like in figure. (see Ep. Lung area and the inferior crus of the helix). | Various kinds of dermal diseases, gynecologic diseases, poor functions of absorption compensation and constipation, etc. |

Table 7–2 Pathological Reactions of Common Diseases on the Auricle

Disease	Region	Reaction
Acute gastritis	Stomach area	Spots or reddish furfurs with luster.
Chronic gastritis	Stomach area	White furfurs with woolly border, mostly, the skin grows thicker (hypertrophic gastritis).
Chronic gastritis in sudden onset	Stomach area	(a) White furfurs or white spots with lustrous redish border. (b) Spots or furfurs with reddishborder or congestion.
Gastric ptosis	Stomach area	Protuberant white furfurs with woolly border at the lateral margin of the stomach area near to the antihelix.
Gastric ulcer	Stomach area	(a) White spots with clear boder. (b) white or dark gray spots with reddishborder; generally all are lustrous. (See Diagram 8–b)
Duodenal ulcer	Duodenum	idem

Chronic enteritis	Large and small intestinal areas	Furfurs or congestive papules, with fat much.
Constipation	Large and small intestinal areas	White furfurs or furfuraceous desquamation, no luster.
Acute appendicitis	Appendix area	Congestive spots or congestive papules.
Choronic appendicitis	Appendix area	The majority appear depressed spots or protuberent spots; The few appear white or dark-gray in colour.
Chronic appendicitis in sudden onset	Appendix area	White spots with reddish border or reddish furfurs.
Acute hepatitis	Liver area	(a) Reddish furfurs or reddish spots. (b) Reddish border with a white center, generally, they are lustrous.
Hepatomegalia	Liver area	Protuberant white furfurs (as a half of a water melon seed) with clear border (if it appears on the right ear that the right lobe of the liver is enlargement; while it appears on the left ear that the left lobe of the liver is enlargement). (See Diagram 8-a.)
Splenomegaly	Spleen area	White furfurs or with reddish border, the few are protuberant.

Disease	Region	Reaction
Pulmonary tuberculosis: Active stage	Lung area	Spots or congestive papules with luster. A few of them to be wiped with a cotton ball will cause bleeding. (If it appears at the lower area, the same side; the upper area, the opposite side).
Calcium stage	Lung area	One to several needle-like depression.
Acute pneumonia	Between both lungs	Redish spots or papules, some of them are white spots with lustrous reddish border.
Acute trachitis	Trachae	Redish spots or papules, few of them are white spots with lustrous reddish border.
Chronic trachitis	Trachae	White spots or furfurs with clear border, a few of them are white papules. All are no luster.
Chronic trachitis in sudden onset	Trachae	White spots or white furfurs, or papules, with reddish border. All are lustrous.
Pulmonary emphysema	Lung area	White furfurs or spots gathering closely as a slice, with a woolly border, but luster during the duration of disease.

Dreams, Insomnia, Erythmia, Extrasystole	Heart area	Circular plice with a luster in the center, a few of them are with a white center.
Rheumatoid cardiopathy	Heart area	White furfurs with woolly border, a few of them are lustrous.
Various kinds of headache and vertigo	Brain spot, brain stem, forehead, subcortex.	Reddish spots or white spots with reddish border, the many are lustrous.
Hypertension	Brain, spot, brain stem, forehead, subcortex.	The reactive regions noted here are the same as those of headache and vertigo. In addition, if Ep, Adrenal gland appears reddish spots or reddish furfurs and Ep. Heart area appear a circular plice, there are white spots or reddish border on 1/3 above Ep, Depressing groove that indicates the systolic pressure of about 150 or so; otherwise if there are reactions in the 1/3 middle of Ep. Depressing groove it indicates the systolic pressure of about 200 or so.
Hypotension	Brain. spot, Brain stem, Forehead, Subcortex.	The reaction of auricular points on the head is the same as that of Ep. Hypertension. If Ep. Adrenal gland has no reaction and there are white spots or reddish border at 1/3 below Ep. Depressing groove, that is hypotension.

Disease	Region	Reaction
Acute sprain of joint	Corresponding region	Reddish spots or reddish furfurs.
Old arthritis	Corresponding region	White spots or reddish furfurs.
Chronic arthritis in sudden onset	Corresponding region	White spots with reddish border, all are lustrous.
Vertebral transformation or Hypertrophic fracture	Corresponding region	Protuberant or protuberant nodules. A few of them are depressed cords in all directions.
Hemorrhoids	Hemorrhoid spot, Lower segment of the rectum	White spots or white furfurs with reddish border. A few of them are dark-gray spots or dark-gary furfurs.
Anal fissure	Hemorrhoid spot, Anus.	White spots with a geel-whell-like reddish border. A few of them are redish spots, as a radiation in figure.
Benign tumor	Corresponding region	Protuberant subcutaneous nodules with clear border, no tenderness. It can remove if pushing.

Malignant tumor	Corresponding region	(a) Protuberant cortilages with woolly border, no removing. (b) A few of them are white or dark-gray furfurs, with marked tenderness.
Dysmenorrhea	Uterus area	White or reddish spots with fat
Hylymenorrhea and Leukorrhea	Uterus area	Dotted congestive papules. (See Diagram 8–b).
Hypomenorrhea or temporary amenorrhea	Uterus area	White spots or white furfurs, no luster; a few of them are furfuranceous desquamation.
Neurodermatitis	Corresponding area to the lung	Furfuranceous desquamation is not easy to be wiped out. (See Diagram 8–b).
Chronic urticaria.	Corresponding to the Lung area	idem
Eczema	Corresponding to the Lung area.	Furfuranceous desquamation is not easy to be wiped out.
Sebothoica dermatitis	Whole auricle	The same as above but with fat.
Scale dermatitis	Whole auricle	Dryness, no luster with scales-like standing up.

Disease	Region	Reaction
Dysfunction of absorption	Whole auricle	Dryness and desquamation, no luster.
All kinds of postoperations	Corresponding region	White shallow triation or semicircle scar, a few of them are in dark-gray colour.
Contraceptives per os	Uterus, Cavum conchae, Symba conchae, Internal secretion	White furfurs desquamation, as a layer of scale-head.

(III) "Pien-cheng" diagnosis of inspection on the auricle

In the process of inspection on the auricle, the characteristics of "a disease has more reactions" and "one point reactes upon more diseases" should be observed seriously.

1. Spot, reddish furfur or congestion (some of them with a reddish border of red papule with fat and luster) usually appear in diseases of acute inflammation.

2. White spot or furfur, depression, protuberance and white papule (all have neither fat nor luster) usually appear in chronic orgainc diseases.

3. Protuberant nodule or dark-gray spot and furfur usually appear in tumor.

4. Furfuraceous desquamation (not easy to be wiped out) usually appears in various kinds of dermal diseases or diseases of the compensatory and obsorbent dysfunction.

5. Stripe-shape, round or semicircle white scar or dark-gray scar usually appear in various kinds of postoperation and scar from wound.

Taking into consideration from several points mentioned above, we have recognized that the reactions of diseases on the auricle have their general regularity. We cannot but grasp the characteristic of the general and the specific, and "a disease has more reactions", and "one point reactes upon more diseases" then combine the clinical symptoms to bring together and analyse them, after that we will be able to make out a initial pien-cheng diagnosis. For instance, laryngitis and tonsillitis all have reactions on a same area (Ep. Tonsil 4). The reactive characteristic of laryngitis appears several white or redish spots with woolly border, while the reactive characteristic of tonsillitis appears reddish furfur or congestion with clear border. Most of these two kinds of inflammation have different reactions on Ep. Tonsil.

(IV) Precautions

1. Observation must be paid carefully to the patient's skin which varies in summer and winter. The skin of an elder person is alos nto the same as that of a child. We should pay more attention to these individual distinction.

2. Before observation, do not wipe, wash, lift or pull the auricle to avoid causing the discoloration of the skin or even wiping out the positive reaction masses that will great influence the accuracy of the inspection. If the depression of the auricle is not clean, may wipe it out lightly along a certain direction with a cotton ball.

3. When the positive reaction is found, the theory of Tsang-fu in Chinese traditional medicine should be taken into consideration, and then carry on comprehensive analysis by the "pien-cheng" method to make out a diagnosis.

4. On the auricle of healthy persons there often appear different manifestations, such as pigementation white nodule, small pustule and scar from pernio, etc. Most of them are "false appearance". A method of distinction: first, to inspect; secondly, to press. No pain when being pressed indicates that it belongs to a "false positive reaction".

5. The light should be sufficient, and the natural light will be the most ideal one; while a flash-light light may also be used by night.

(V) Realization of the inspection on the auricle

In the clinical practice we have had some initial realization concerning the inspection on the auricle:

1. Through the inspection of the auricle, we have gone a step further in recognizing the localization of auricular points. For example, the pathological reaction of hemiplegia, osteohyperplasia of spine and prolapse of lumbar intervestebral disk are at the high point of the antihelix but not at the medial margin of the antihelix;and as Ep Lung (located in the cavum conchae of the auricle) is divided into two areas: the lower area is the lung of the same side, while the upper one is that of the opposite side.

2. Through the inspection of the auricle, the therapeutic effect of the ear acupuncture has been increased. If prick the needle exactly into the pathological reaction spot being inspected. the result is better.

3. Through the inspection of the auricle, our knowledge of the "Pien-cheng" of Tsang-fu in Chinese traditional medicine has gone a step further. Those such as "The heart controls the mind and the spirit", dreams, insomnia and diseases of the nervous and mental system are all having their reactions at Ep.Heart area. "The spleen and the stomach are connected with each other and as the interior-exterior relationships", so diseases of chronic gastritis, gastric or duodenal ulcer and indigestion (poor in transportation), have their reactions at the Ep. Stomach area as the same at the Ep. Spleen area. "The lung controls the skin and hair", hence all kinds of dermal diseases have their reactions at Ep. Lung area, etc. We find conform to the theory of Tsang-fu.

4. The inspection of the auricle has exhibited a new way of initial and differential diagnosis of some diseases such as tumor, acute appendicitis, etc., which deserves to be further searched out.

What mentioned above are some ideas obtained in the

practice of the auricular inspection. Although the characteristic diagnosis of some maladies can be made, yet of the
majority of diseases, only the illness appeared in the corresponding regions are known. Therefore, the conclusion should
not be drawn from the auricular inspection only; we should
make a concrete analysis of concrete problems.

Chapter VIII

METHODS OF USING A DETECTOR

AND ANALYSIS OF SENSITIVE SPOTS

(I) Methods of Using a Detector

1. When turn on the "power switch" of the apparatus, an earphone (loudspeaker) gives forth a buzzing sound like, "wong, wong, wong!" (1,000 Hz. or so).

Plunge the plug of the text probe into the "ditector socket", by this time if the sound disappears, it indicates that the apparatus is normal.

2. Holding a test probe (i.e. electrode) in one hand, the practitioner use another hand to put and press another probe tightly on the patient's Pt. Neikuan-68 (P 6)--the test probe had best be tightened with an electro-band of the ECG--then press the end of the test probe on the patient's Pt. Hoku-84 (LI 4) or Ep. Spinal cord (on the auricle), adust the sensivity of the "potentio-meter" slowly to cause the earphone to give forth a certain sound, the volume of the sound may be controlled by the user himself, while the user should bear the loudness of the sound in mind.

During detection, the place that gives forth such a sound is a sensitive spot; otherwise it is a negative one; while the appearance of the sound with a tingle in the detected area shows that the spot is a strong positive spot.

3. Write down the reactive condition of every sensitive spot according to the following symbols. Now, let us take Ep. Kidney as an example:

K (Ep. Kidney): write down only an auricular point without any symbols, indicating there occurs a sound.

K There occurs not only a sound but also a stinging feeling — a strong positive one.

K* There occurs a sound, but a light one.

K There is no sound, but the patient has a stinging feeling or tenderness.

4. Two methods of examination are as follows:

(a) Examine each point of the auricle one by one from above downward. Generally points of the internal organs at first; then the trunk; finally four limbs (i.e. Eps. Cymba conchae, Cavum conchae, triangular fossa; the antihelix, helix, auricular lobute, scapha and the back of the auricle). It requires more careful examination of each area concerned refering to symptoms of which the patient himself complains.

(b) Examination according to the system: In using the method, the practitioner should be quite familiar with the reaction law of every kinds of illness appearing on the uaricle. After a sensitive spot is found out, all the corresponding which have relation with the spots and may cause diseases should be examined. If it agrees with fact, we may make a tentative diagnosis and then go on with further examination. For instance, in examining a case, if we find that the patient's Ep. Gallbladder area presents a strong positive reaction (GB), we should make a further examination of the Eps. Liver, Shoulder joint and Lateral abdomen; the appearance of sensitive spots presented by these points shows that it is possible that the patient is suffering from cholecystitis; if there are no such three points, but only a reaction with a light sound on Ep. Liver area (LV),thus the appearance of the sensitive spot may be caused by liver disease. By this time we should exclude cholecystitis first, and then examine carefully the concerning points which are connected with the diseases of the liver system. This method is suitable for the differential diagnosis.

5. Methods of manipulation

The changes of sensitive spots of the auricle differ from one another, depending upon the patient's age, sex, condition of work, the kind and the extent of diseases, the climate, surroundings, temperature and the moisture capasity, etc. At the same time they have close relation to the properties of apparatus and the methods of manipulation.

The properties of the apparatus mostly depend upon the design and the manufacture of the apparatus. As to the method of manipulation, we hold that a light manipulation is applied generally on the cavum conchae, cymba conchae, auricular lobute, triangular fossa and the scapha, where the skin is soft; while the stronger one is applied on the antihelix and antitragus. Within the same area, the distinction of the sensitive points should be made by comparing them with each other under the condition of concerted manipulation.

6. When the examination is done, take away the "test probe" and the "earphone ",then turn off the power.

7. The voltage of the dry battery used in the apparatus will influence the sensitivity greatly. Generally battery of 9V is to be used, but when the voltage becomes lesser than 8V, it should not be used again.

(II) A Comprehensive Analysis on Detection
Results of Sensitive Spots

In the process of detecting the sensitive spots of the auricle, a disease constantly presents several sensitive spots, while a sensitive spot is also communized by many diseases, their relations are more complicated. Provided that we combine these sensitive spots earnestly with patient's ill history, and make a comprehensive induction and analysis, we should get a more precise judgement in the distinction of the disease.

An ordinary analysis depends upon three aspects:
1. The theory of Tsang-fu* is the theory of studying physiologic functions, pathological changes and their interrelations in Chinese tradional medicine. In the process of detecting auricular points, it is more valuable for reference in using the theory of Tsang-fu to explain the reason of why some sensitive spots appear, sum-up and diagnose these sensitive spots, and use the results to guide medical practice. As in a case of fracture, apart from the sensitive spots

*The theory of Tsang Fu
The meaning of Tsang Fu indicates on the one hand the organs which can be seen with the naked eyes; on the other hand also a summing up of the physiological functions and pathological changes of these organs. Therefore there is a certain distinction between the Tsang Fu of Chinese traditional medicine and the idea of internal organs of modern medical science; these two ideas should not be confused. In the theory of Tsang Fu, the internal organs are divided into two large categories of Tsang and Fu. Tsang includes the heart, the liver, the spleen, the lungs, and kidneys, called the five Tsang, in addition also the outer surrounding of the heart (circulation sex), altogether called the six Tsang. Fu, includes the small intestine, the gall-bladder, the stomach, the large intestine, the urinary bladder and the triple wormer, altogether called the six Fu. The brain, the cerebral fluid and the womb are otherwise called "Chi heng chih fu". Different Tsang Fu, each has a different function, furthermore it has a mutual relationship and a mutual influence.

appearing on the corresponding areas of the auricle, in accordance with the theory of "The kidney governs the bone" in Chinese traditional medicine, generally there can also appear sensitive spots on Ep. Kidney area of the auricle. And when the lung suffered from organic diseases, in addition to Ep. Lung area appearing a marked sensitive reaction, ordinarily the sensitive spots can also appear on the Ep. Large intestine area in accordance with the theory of "The lung and the large intestine are connected with each other, forming the internal-external relationship" in Chinese traditional medicine. Furthermore, during detection, if Eps. Heart, Shenmen and Subcortex appear sensitive spots, we should take them into consideration that the sensitive reactions appear not only on the Ep. Heart area of the auricle, but also on Ep. Small intestine. If there is no sensitive spot appearing on the Ep. Small intesine area, generally the possibilty of diseases of the heart may be excluded, it may be insomnia, palpitation or other symptoms caused by "The heart and the kidney are not discord with each other". Such a analytical method is most frequently applied in the clinical practice.

2. Analysis according to the theory of modern medicine:

For instance, in the case of duodenal ulcer, the patient's Ep. Duodenum detected presents a sensitive spot. In terms of anatomy, the duodenum is controlled by the vegetative nerve, and the pain caused by duodenal ulcer is bound to involve the changes of sympathetic nerve. Therefore, the sensitive spot usually appears on Ep. Sympathy of the patient's auricle; while the pain caused from duodenal ulcer is mostly radiating to the back side. Hence the sensitive spot may appear on the Ep. Lumbo-sacral area. Furthermore, In accordance with the theory "Ulcerative diseases is caused by the disturbance of central function of the subcortex", it may be reasoned out that sensitive spots may usually appear on

Eps. Subcortex and Shenmen on the auricle of the patient with duodenal ulcer.

3. Analysis according to reference points of various kinds of diseases:

For certain diseases having been accurately diagnosed, it is necessary to detect auricular points carefully in more cases, write down the sites of every sensitive spots in detail. After statistics, select several auricular points (usually 3-5 points) which the appearance-rate of the sensitive spots is higher. We may preliminarily hold that when these auricular points appearing sensitive spots must have a definite relation with certain diseases. Therefore, in making a comprehensive analysis, we regard these points as "the reference points for diagnosis of certain diseases". For instance in 52 accurately diagnosed cases of nephritis, we detected the sensitive spots on the patients' auricle, and found out their distribution as shown on Table 8-1.

The table shows that on Eps. Kidney, Urinary bladder, Internal secretion and Nephritis spot, of the 52 cases of nephritis, the appearance of the sensitive spots is as high as 51 cases. This gives an illustration of the fact that the above four sensitive spots have certain relation with nephritis, so we call them "Reference points for diagnosis of nephritis".

For various kinds of diseases, we should make a lot of detection on the auricular points separately, so as to enable us to grasp some rules gradually. In using this method, the obtained reference points for diagnosis would be more valuable if a certain quantity of contrasting detection is made at the same time (e.g. contrast the case of nephritis with the case of non-nephritis).

The reference points for diagnosis of common diseases are now listed in the following table for further discussion.

Table 8—1 The Distributed Condition of Auricle-Sensitive Spots on 52 Patients with Nephritis

Eps.	Kidney	Urinary bladder	Internal secretion	Nephritis spot	Ureter	Sanchiao	Shoulder joint	Sympathy	Stomach	Liver
R.A.*	52	51	52	52	25	27	31	17	31	11

Eps.	Esophagus	Lumbago spot	Ear-Shenmen	Occiput	Uterus	Adrenal gland	Heart	Trachae	Mouth	Eye
R.A.	47	43	51	24	19	19	21	19	21	11

Eps.	Large intestine
R.A.	21

* Rate of appearance

Table 8-2 The Reference Points for Diagnosis of Some Common Diseases

Order number	Disease	Primary point	Auxiliary point	Remarks
1	Hepatitis	Hepatitis area: Hepatitis spot.	Internal secretion; Sympathy	
		Kanyang 1; kanyang 2.		The function of liver may be abnormal
2	Hepatomegalia	Hepatomegalia area; Sanchiao.		often appear on the right ear
3	Schistosomiasis	Sensitive line of schistosome.	Large intestine.	often appear on the right ear
4	Cholecystitis	Gallbladder; lateral abdomen.	Stomach; Liver; Shoulder.	often appear on the right ear
5	Appendicitis	Appendix	Large intestine; Sanchiao.	often appear on the right ear

		Points of the corresponding area.		at both sides
6	Hypertrophic spinitis		Kidney	
7	Nephretis	Kidney; Nephritis spot	Urinary bladder; Internal secretion	same as above
8	Pyelonephritis	Nephritis spot; External genital organs; Urethra; Kidney.	Urinary bladder; Internal secretion.	same as above
9	Constipation	Constipation spot	Large intestine	same as above
10	Hemorrhoids	Constipation spot; Lower segment of the rectum	Large intestine; Sanchiao.	same as above
11	Neurasthenia	Subcortex; Shenmen	Heart	same as above
12	Mammitis	Thorax; Mammary gland	Internal secretion	often appear on at the same side
13	Asthma	Bronchi	Asthma spot; Soothing asthma	
14	Hepatic cirrhosis	Muscular flaxation spot; Hepatomegalia area.	Stomach; Esophagus	

Order number	Disease	Primary point	Auxiliary point	Remarks
15	Sexual involution in male	Testicle, Uterus	Excitement spot	
16	Gastritis	Stomach; Esophagus	Orifice; Small intestine.	

Supplemental diagram: Detection of blood pressure

Upper

Middle

Lower

Depressing groove

Systolic pressure

Diastolic pressure

Point for lowering blood pressure

Point for raising blood pressure

Supplemental table: Reaction of Reference points for Diagnosis of Blood Pressure

Estimation of the measurement of blood pressure	Point for raising blood pressure	Point for lowering blood pressure	Depressing groove		
			Upper	Middle	Lower
90/60 mm Hg ± 5	+	—	+	—	—
130/ 90 mm Hg ± 5	+	+	±	—	+
140/ 100 mm Hg ± 5	±	+	++	—	±
150/ 110 mm Hg ± 5	++	+	++	—	±
180/ 120 mm Hg ± 5	++	++	+	++	+

Notes: +: sound
±: sound with tingling
++: higher sound
±±: high sound with tingling

Case Reports or Recommendable Case Reports

Case 1.

Hsu xx, male, age 64.

Complaints: Hematemesis attacked in a sudden half a month ago, asphalt-like stool accompanied with dizziness, blurred vision and fatigue, neither abdominal pain, nor past history of stomachalgia.

A record of detection of sensitive spots:

Right auricle: Eps. Uterus, Stomach, Cardiac orifice, Subcortex, Internal secretion, Adrenal gland, A segment of Tonsil 4 ~ Helix 4, Heart, Occiput, Mouth and Esophagus.

Analysis in Conjunction with the case history:

Asphalt-like stool and hematemesis indicate bleeding in the upper digestive tract and the tingling is obvious when Eps. Stomach and Cardiac orifice is detected. From this we further confirm that the patient falls ill in the digestive system. No history of stomachalgia-anamnesis, and no sensitive spots on Eps. Sympathy and Lumba-sacral vertebra indicate the remote possibility of chronic ulcer. In addition, a feeling of tingling in sensitive spots Eps. Internal secretion, Subcortex, Adrenal gland and a line of Tonsil 4~Helix 4 indicate that the probability is that the case is of malignat tumor located between the cardiac orifice and the stomach area.

According to the detection of auricular points in conjunction with the case history, we deduce that the posibility is that the case is of cancer of stomach or cancer of cardiac orifice.

Thereafter a barium meal examination of the patient's gastro-intestinal tract was made by the No. 2 Hospital attached to the Nanking New medical College and confirmed the diagnosis of cancer of esophagus-cardiac orifice in the gastric basis.

Case 2.

Fan xx, male, age 34.

The patient asked for a physical examination to see whether he had any ailment or not, and was eager to know the accuracy of diagnosing diseases by means of the detector.

A record of detection of sensitive spots:

Eps. Shenmen, Subcortex, Point of lowering blood pressure +, Point of raising blood pressure +, the upper segment of Depressing groove +, the lower segment of Depressing groove +, Bronchitis spot, Pharynx-Larynx, Sympathy, Stomach, Occiput, Shoulder joint, Toothache spot, Anesthesis for extraction of teeth, Sanchiao, Constipation spot, Large intestine, Lumbago spot and Esophagus.

Inductive analysis according to the reaction of sensitive spot: The emergence of sensitive spots on Subcortex and Shenmen is mostly caused by pain, while the emergence of sensitive spots on Eps. Sympathy, Sanchiao, Stomach and Esophagus accompanied with a slight tingling in Ep. Stomach indicates the fact that the pain has relations with stomach area, thus we deduce that there is a great possibility of being gastritis.

Analysis of Eps. Point of lowering blood pressure +, Point of raising blood pressure +, the upper segment of Depressing groove +, and the lower segment of Depressing groove + in conjunction with referring to Table 8-2, it indicates that the patient's blood pressure is around 130/90 mm Hg.

The emergence of sensitive spots on Eps. Toothache spot and Anesthesia for extraction of teeth at the same time indicates that the pain is possibly caused by ginivitis, pulpitis, decayed teeth, or tooth defect, ect.

The emergence of sensitive spots on Eps. Constipation spot, large intestine, The sun, Forehead and Lumbago spot indicates that the patient by this time has the symptoms of dry stool, dizziness, sore loins, etc. Analysis of the sensitive spots of Eps. Bronchitis spot and Pharynx-Larynx in conjunction with the sensitive spots of Eps. Sympathy and Shenmen: Pharyngitis and bronchitis may be deduced. But the feeling of tingling in Eps. Bronchitis and Pharynx-Larynx, and the changes of the skin are not obvious, thus the patient has suffered from inflammation for a long time. Which is likely chronic inflammation.

Initial impression:	(a) Blood pressure 130/ 90 mm Hg.;
	(b) Chronic gastritis;
	(c) Chronic pharyngitis, chronic bronchitis;
	(d) Toothache or tooth defect;
	(e) Dry stool, dizziness, sore loins, etc.
Past illness:	(a) In 1958, the patient suffered from stomach disease constantly with acid regurgitation, lack of appetite. Barium meal examination had been made many times but there was not any abnormality being found. In addition, he has suffered from trachitis for many years, frequently with coughing. (b) Before detection, the blood pressure was 128/ 90 mm Hg. (c) Other symptoms were basically in confirmity with the result of the auricular detection.

Case 3.

Zhu xx, female, age 41.

She asked for a detection of auricular points to diagnose her illness.

A record of detection of sensitive spots:

    Right auricle: Eps. Uterus, Shenmen, Point of lowering blood pressure−, Hepatitis spot, Hepatitis area, Kidney, Sympathy, Hepatomegaly area, Lung area, Internal secretion, External genital organs, Kanyang 1, Point of raising blood pressure +, the upper segment of Depressing groove +, Esophagus, Stomach, lumbago spot, Sanchiao, Shoulder joint, Pelvic cavity and Subcortex.

Inductive analysis of sensitive spots:

    On detection, if there are more sensitive spots, they should be inductively classified and gradually analysed. In this case, The emergence of sensitive spots on five Eps. Hepatitis area, Kanyang 1, Hepatitis spot, Internal secretion and Sympathy at the same time indicates that there is an inflammation in the liver. But Eps. Kanyang 2 and Asites have no reaction sheds light on the transformation of hepatitis to a chronic stage, with normal functioning power of the liver.

    The sensitive spot of Eps. Hepatomegaly area and the middle of the lower area of the right auricle indicate hepatomegaly (infracosta) about 2.5 cm.

    The emergence of sensitive spots on Eps. Stomach and Esophagus indicates that the liver and the stomach are discordant, uncomforatble in the stomach and abdominal distention caused by chronic hepatitis.

    Eps. Subcortex, Shenmen and Sanchiao may be considered as the reaction of the pain in the liver area. The emergence of sensitive spots on Eps. Uterus, External genital organs and Pelvic cavity is usually caused by gynecologic diseases. In this case, it is quite within the bound of possibility that the disease is cervicitis. As to the sensitive spots emerge on the bronchial site of Ep. Lung area, the patient has no feeling of tingling, thus it may be an ailment of chronic bronchitis.

In the case of hepatitis, the symptom of dizziness usually has a reaction of sensitive spots on Eps. Forehead and The sun, only rarely sensitive spots emerge on Ep. Lumbago. The patient told us that she had sprained her waist once and still had a symptom of lumbago.

Past illness, physical examination and some specific examina tion:

Complaints: Hepatitis for 12 years; in 1969, she suffered from viral pneomonia; at present, she still has coughing once in a while, and leukorrhagia.

Physical examination: Blood pressure 96/58 mm Hg. Hepatomegaly (infracosta) 2-3 cm., the pain attacks during a light percution or palpation.

Liver function: Normal

Supersonic wave: Liver (infracosta) 2.5 cm.

Case 4.

Li xx, female, age 69.

Chief complaints: Abdominal pain, sometimes seriously, disliked food, bedridden for a week.

A tentative examination made by another hosiptal, consideration:

(a) Acute gastritis? (b) Cancer of stomach? Thereafter, the patient was transferred to our hospital and received an examination of sensitive spots of the auricle.

A record of detection of sensitive spots:

Eps. Gallbladder, Liver, Stomach, Abdomen, Occiput, Internal secretion, Sympathy, Shenmen, Subcortex and Lateral abdomen.

Comparative analysis referring to the ill history and the results of the tentative examination made by another hospital and combined with the record of detection of suricular points:

The sensitive spots of the patient with gastriris are mostly on the areas of Eps. Esophagus, Cardiac orifice, Stomach, Duodenum on the pheriperal crus of the helix.

The patient has a pain in the abdomen and dislikes food, it generally has an ailment in the digestive system. having relation with the stomach area. But the sensitive spot emerges on Ep. Gallbladder when it is detected, also the tingling reaction is stronger than that of Ep. Stomach area. In accordance with the statistic data of cholecystitis by detecting auricular points, such a condition indicated that the cause of the patient's abdominal pain is possibly caused by cholecystitis, and not gastritis.

patient's snesitive spots, we hold that the patient possibly have cancer of stomach.

After analysis of the reaction or the patient's sensitive spots, we hold that it is quite not possible that she is suffering from cancer of stomach.

In July 3, 1971, according to the clinical observation and test combined with the gallbladder radiography by Shanghai Rui-Chin Hospital, the final diagnosis was chronic cholecystitis in acute onset.

Chapter IX

" SELECTION OF POINTS

BY THE PIEN-CHENG" METHOD

IN PRACTICAL USE

Selection of points by the "pien-cheng" method* is the most important. In the process of treatment. Whether the embodiment is correct or not has great influence on the transformation of diseases; correct embodiment will give a good therapeutic result, otherwise the result is bad, or even invalid.

Once we treated a patient suffered from gastric ulcer for four years. In his gastric region occured a hungry pain for quite some time, he had poor appetite, we found that having taken plentiful meal, he felt uncomfortable in the stomach, while just a moment after taking a pitance of food felt a pain in his stomach accompained by abdominal distention.

By this time, his face was pale, his limbs were weak. Through diagnoses done in many hospitals, physicians all considered that the patient had to be operated. But he did not agree with it, he asked for ear acupuncture treatment

---

*Selection of Points by the pien-cheng method in Chinese traditional medicine:
    Points are selected according to the Pien-cheng method in Chinese traditional medicine, i.e. first distinguish the relationships between the symptoms of disease or the responses of the patient during treatment and the Tsang-fu and Ching-lo, and then determine the involved points according to the principles of Tsang-fu functions and their interrelations.
    This method is usually used in co-ordination with other concept.

instead of it.

Gastric ulcer is a kind of common disease due to the ailment in the digestive tract, so we applied a symtomatic treatment according to the patient's main symptom.

Selected points: Sympathy, Shenmen, Stomach, Subcortex.

After three treatments, the patient reflected that the pain was reduced, his appetite improved, and we found him on a fair towards recovery from abdominal distention. Thereafter, the disease was not stable. After persisting in three courses of the treatment, 32 treatments in all, although some painful symptoms have been relaxed and controlled, the disease still could not be cured fundamentally. The patient encouraged us to give further treatment. We held that some symptoms have been relaxed and controlled, besides the subjective symptoms were improving, such as a change on his face from pale into tender and rosy, fowerful in movement of his limbs—these themselves were pregnant with the curing factors. Then, according to the symptoms, making reference to knowledge of such a diseases in Chinese traditional and Western medicine, the patient, together with us, analysed the diary of the previous 32 treatments. We held that the above assorted point-prescription was only for symptomatic treatment, short of treatment by "p i en-cheng sih chih" *. We made up a new prescription in accordance with the principle of treatment in Chinese traditional medicine: "Increase the function of the spleen and help the stomach", "Build up the normal, and wipe away the abnormal".

Selected points: Shenmen, Sympathy, Stomach, Spleen and Lung. The former prescription was mainly for symptomatic treatment, just the same as from selection of points to the manipulation, so the patient felt only some relaxation of general symptom; while the later prescription seized hold of the principal contradiction, mainly for strengthening the spleen, by applying strong stimulation of one point with more needles inserted in Ep. Spleen, and applying weak stimulation in Ep. Stomach.

After three treatments, stomachalgia and abdominal distention disappeared, the patient's appetite was marked improving; and after 14 treatments, X – rayed examination showed that the ulcer as large as an almond within the lesser gastric curvature formerly existing disappeared. The patient's health was restored. Why, could we obtain therapeutic effect by changing a few points? we held that it has seized the main aspects of contradiction—"Strengthening the spleen" depending upon the "pien-cheng sih chih" in Chinese traditional medicine.

In the process of treating disease of gastric ulcer, we had

---

*"Pien-Cheng Sih Chih"

Human body is a united whole of contradictions, every part of the body physiologically keeps in close connection with one another. After the onset of diseases, the local ailment is bound to have an affection on other parts as well as the whole, while the transformation of the whole will certainly exert an influence upon the local. Therefore, in the course of clinical diagnosis and treatment, the relation between the local and the whole should be handled judiciously.

"Pien-cheng" means to distinguish "Cheng hou"—both subjective and objective symptoms manifested by diseases. "Cheng hou" consists of many concrete symptoms, it is not equivalent to a simple array of symptoms, but analysis, anthesis and induction of symptoms, with discarding the dross and selecting the essential, eliminating the false and retaining the trus, proceeding from one to the other and from the outside to the inside to form the systems of conception and theory by which the interrrelation among the symptoms, the cause of diseases, the sites of ailments as well as their pathological changes are found; thus finally drawn is the conception of "Cheng hou", serving as the basis of treatment. In a word, what so called symptoms are only the phenomenon of diseases, offering data for "Pien-cheng", while "Pien cheng" means to grasp the essence of disease by distinguishing the symptoms.

"Sih chih"—a term in Chinese traditional medicine that means to set a therapeutic method according to the principles of curing diseases in Chinese traditional, medicine after analysing and synthesizing the symptoms of the patient's disease.

deepened our knowledge and apprehension of selection of points by "pien-cheng" method and also realized and found out some dialectical relationship between the application of assorted points-prescription according to the different diseases and the acupuncture manipulation.

One more example:

A patient suffered from chronic dysentery for more than ten years, had abdominal distention, abnormal in bowel movement and was losing his appetite and emaciated all the year round. He had been sent to hospital several times, once for over two years.

The patient had taken various kinds of drugs, received many methods of treatments, but his illness could not be cured basically. Routine examination of stool, red cell ++, pus cell ++~+++, and stool cultivation were positive. We were lack of clinical experience of curing this chronic disease. Under the close co-ordination of the patient, we decided to cure the symptoms of abdominal distention and abdominal pain first. Assorted points-prescription: Sympathy, Shenmen, Large intestine, Small intestine and Abdomen. After a course of treatment, it got only some relaxation of pain, but the therapeutic effect was less satisfactory. We studied the therapeutic condition of using the above-mentioned prescription in co-ordination with patient's ill history and held that since he had chronic dysentery for such a long time, that the intestinal mucosa of large intestine was found in chronic ulcer and edema, rather difficult to heal up, and also on account of tolerating drug-treatment, this chronic disease was not easy to get a good result in a short period. In the light of diagnosis and clinical experiences in Chinese traditional and Western medicine,   we took away Eps. Abdomen and Shenmen from the Prescription as noted above (according to clinical experience, sometimes, it will increase abdominal distention if Ep. Shenmen is inserted), add Eps. Lung and Heart (because the theory of Tsang-fu tells us that the lung and the large intestine are connected with each other, forming the unternal–external relationship", and so the heart and the small intestine. Practice has proved that needling Ep. Lung gives a comparatively good curative effect for ulcer. Thus after twice of treatments, the patient reflected that his abdominal pain and abdominal distention disappeared, while his appetite was good after ten treatments, the stool cultivation turned into negative. To consolidate the therapeutic result, we continued it with a course of treatment, and eventually, such a chronic dysentery lasting for ten years was basically cured.

Selection of points by the "pien-cheng" method is that, according to the "pien-cheng" of "Tsang-fu" in Chinese traditional medicine, we have come to know the symptom appearing in the patient from all sides; by analysing and clarifying the reason why the disease has appeared, the region the nature and the cause of disease, and its course of development to grasp the essense of illness and then determine the point prescription seriously. On the prescription, the relation between the primary and auxiliary points should be handled correctly. The emergence and development of disease are the result of contradictory strugle and transformation in the human organism. Human body is a united whole, the cerebrum, peripheral nerves, internal organs and four limbs are all interconnected and interacted with one another. The accurrence of any disease is not isolated, there must be a pair of principal contradiction playing a decisive action, while some others are the secondary contradictions. A common saying: "In studying any complex process in which there are two or more contradictions, we must devote every effort to finding its principal contradiction. Once this principal contradiction is gasped, all problems can be really solved." Selection of points by the pien-cheng method in ear acupuncture is aiming at finding out the relation between focus and organism, finding out the principal and the secondary contradictions and holding them properly, giving the right treatment against the disease in order to recover the patient's health.

Concerning the basis of selection of points for ear acupuncture, we have an primilinary realization of three methods:
1. Selection of points according to the corresponding area.

This is a method in accordance with sensitive spots and tenderness on the auricle reflected by diseases of internal organs and limbs. As in stomachalgia, needle the sensitive spots of Ep. Stomach (the area where the disappearance of the crus of the helix); In fracture of the clavicle, Ep. Clavicle on the scapha may be inserted, etc. All of these are the applications of the method of the selection of points according to the corresponding area. It is a more effective method for some acute diseases.

2. Selection of points by the "pien-cheng" method in Chinese traditional medicine. The application of the theory of Tsang-fu in the clinical practice of ear-acupuncture has led us to avoid making mistakes. A great deal of practice has proved the scientific character of the theory. For instance, the internal external relationship between the heart and the small intestine; the lung and the large intestine; the kidney and the urinary bladder, the stomach and the spleen, and the liver and the gallbladder, etc. Although how abstract as they sound, yet the practically therapeutic effect exists subjectively. As in diseases of the cardiovascular system, there appears also reaction on Ep. Small intestine concerned, so if Ep. Small intestine in combined with other points to treat cardiovascular diseases, the therapeutic result will be better.

In cases of indigestion and dysturbance of intestine, if it is combined with Ep. Heart, the therapeutic effect is more satisfactory; and as we use Ep. kidney to treat diseases of tinnitus and otitis media according to the theory "The kidney shows itself on the ear" in Chinese traditional medicine, we will get a marked therapeutic result too.

3. Selection of points according to the function of commonly used points and clinical experience.

The method can be assensed and grasped only by a great deal of clinical practice, otherwise it is unable to take the anitiative in the process of treatment. In addition, in the clinical practice, a few of points should be selected and used accurately. Usually, select points at the affected side, and a limited number of points are selected at the contralateral side, if necessary. For strengthening the therapeutic effect, points at either sides may be applied.

Chapter X

CARE REPORT

1. Duodenal ulcer

Zhang xx, male, age 45.

Zhang had suffered from duodenal ulcer for more than twenty years. The patient's gastro-intestinal barium meal examination by X-rays showed that there emerged an ulcerous shadow as large as an almond in his duodenum. The patient felt a pain in the stomach region and had sour regurgitation after meal every day, especially at midnight, he was unable to endure the pain.

After taking a plentiful meal or something indigestible, the pain was more serious, radiating to the back region. Malnutrition for a long time, insomnia and even asphalt-like stools in recent years had caused the patient to become emaciated day by day.

In the past for more than twenty years, the patient had taken various kinds of drugs and injections, but it was all in vain.

Spring of 1970, the case condition became serious, the patient's stomach region was painful without interruption, the upper digestive tract was bleeding. By this time, the patient required treatment by auriculotherapy.

Selected points: Eps. Sympathy, Ear-Shenmen, Duodenum,

Stomach, Lung and Subcortex.

Initial analysis: Ulcerous pain is constantly irritated by the local focus, so as the stomach and the duodenum usually stand in the spasmodic condition, lead to the abnormality of the blood circulation of the peripheral focus. Chinese traditional medicine takes the view that the pain results from abnormal following motion of the blood and chi (vital energy). Therefore a group of points-prescription noted above is adopted. At first, the pain should be releaved, and then the local nutritional condition should be improved and the function of that organs should be restored too. Thus we select Eps. Sympathy, Shenmen and Subcortex aiming to adjust the function of the vegetative nerve and the cerebral cortex, sedation and relieving the pain.

Eps. Duodenum and Stomach are used to promote the corresponding internal organs，strengthen their capability against diseases and improve their functions so as to reach a new balance. In addition, Ep. Lung is used for the purpose of increasing the curing effect in mucosal ulcer.

After needling the above-mentioned points seven times, the patient felt himself better than before. His sour regurigitation decreased obviously, his stomachalgia disappeared basically. From now then, the patient insisted on four courses of treatments, his subjective symptom was restored thoroughly. X-ray examination confirmed that the patient's ulcer in the duodenal glomerulus was lost to sight.

The patient said, "Since the past more than twenty years, I have never had it so comfortable!"

2. Acute Infectious Hepatitis
Zhu xx, male, age 36.

Having been attacked by fever for 6-7 days without interruption, the patient's had lost his appitite. He hated taking greasy food and was generally feeble. The colour of his skin turned into yellow. The definite diagnosis by a hospital told that it was a infectious hepatitis. The liver function of the patient was abnormal, the S.G.P.T. 300 units.

After being treated under auriculotherapy several times, he felt his fever had been reduced and his appetite increased obviously. After ten treatments, the S.G.P.T. dropped to be 68 unites, the icteric index dropped from 30 to 14 unites. Following the second course of treatment, he felt comfortable all over, his appetite was as good as usual. Reviewing examination showed that the function of his liver was normal. In the duration of treatment, the patient took only a small dose of vitamin, no other drugs had been taken.

Selected points: Eps. Liver, Spleen, Gallbladder, Internal secretion, Sympathy and Kanyang 1-2.

Initial analysis: Use Ep. Liver to control some symptoms caused by infectious hepatitis and asist to restore the action of the hepatic cell. Because "The liver and the gallbladder are connected with each other, forming the internal—external relationship", they have the functions of promoting each other as well as they can decrease the icteric index of icterohepatitis, thus Ep. Gallbladder is selected. And the selection of Ep. Internal secretion is due to making it better for excretion, absorption of organism and improvement of the compensating function.

If this group of auricular points is used in the treatment of other patients with hepatitis, it will get expected effect too.

3. Neurasthenia

Hsing xx, male, age 48.

Having suffered from neurasthenia for twenty years, Hsing was sleepless all night for quite some time. Occationally he slept 3-4 hours, but got mentally confused at the day time.

In the past twenty years, Hsing had never left soporific drugs with him. Hsing's memory was declining, which affected his work and study seriously. In November 1972, Hsing began to receive auriculotherapy.

Selected points: Eps. Heart, Kidney, Subcortex, Shenmen and blood letting on the apex of the auricle.

Initial analysis: The theory of Chinese traditional medicine considers that "The heart stores the mind and controls the blood". Hence the patient has symptoms of fainting and heavy feeling in the brain. "The kidney stores the spirit", its function has closely related with the heart. When "The heart is out of accord with the kidney", there will have a serious symptoms of neurasthenia. Furthermore, "The brain is the mansion of the spirit", being a controller of the activity of the mind, thus we select Eps. Shenmen and Subcortex to regulate the actions of excitement or inhibition of the cerebral cortex in order to cause them to reach a new balance. And blood-letting of the apex of the auricle has a favourable action of sedation and lowering blood pressure.

After the first treatment, Hsing felt sleepy; after the second treatment, he slept 4-5 hours at that night. Until the second course of treatment was over, he slept 6-7 hours each night. In the daytime, Hsing worked vigorously and the symptoms disappeared entirely.

4. Otitis Media

Zhang xx, female, age 19.

The patient told us that she had suffer from purulent in both ears since she was one year old, From now then, her hearing sensation got more and more worse. Since the past 18 years, the pus has been found flowing out from her ears on and on all the year round, it constantly dispersed stink in the summer season.

After five treatments by auriculotherapy, the pus stopped and the inflammation disappeared.

Selected points: Eps. Kidney, External ear, Internal ear, Internal secretion and Occiput.

Initial analysis: Neiching says "The energy of Kidneys is linked with the ears, if the kidneys are mild the ears can hear all sound". It can be perceived that the relation between the kidneys and the ears is very close, this indicates that an ailment in the ears may be cured by dint of strengthening the kidneys, thus Ep. Kidney is selected; while Eps. Internal ear and External ear are used to play a part directly in the local ailment, promoting the local capability of anti diseases to reach a new balance. As to select Eps. Occiput and Internal secretion is in order to eliminate inflammation.

5. Aural Vertigo

Chai xx, female, age 43.

Chai had a four-year case history. When the illness attacked, she was enable to move her head up and open her eyes, she felt fainting seriously with vomiting without interruption. Sometimes, the symptom usually lasted for several weeks. In August 1970, the symptom mentioned above occured again. Three days later Chai began to receive the treatment of ear acupuncture.

Selected points: Eps. Occiput, Shenmen and Stomach are used with the purpose of regulating the activity of the nerve center concerned and controlling the symptoms of vertigo and fainting, also causing the action of stopping vomiting. Since these symptoms generally attach to the labyrinthic internal ear, Ep. Internal ear is used for treating the underlying disease. In the literature of Chinese traditional medicine we can find out the versions of "The brain is a sea of the narrow" and "The energy of the kidneys reaches the ear", which shows   that   the kidneys and the brain as well as   the kidneys and the ears are all connected with each other closely. In the process. of treating this disease,   since Ep. Kidney has been added, the therapeutic effect is obviously increased.

The patient got up and was capable of activity after three treatments and she was cured after seven treatments. A year later the physicians followed up the patient, Chai said,"In the past, the disease would attack several times a year, but since being treated under the auriculo-therapy, it has never attack again up to the present day. How excellent the auriculo-therapy is!"

Appendix 1

AURICULAR POINTS-PRESCRIPTION

USED IN ACUPUNCTURE ANESTHESIA

Supplement: Methods of Acupuncture Anesthesia

Needles be inserted into some definite auricular points to induce analgesia for operation is a main component of acupuncture anesthesia.

Keep it for reference of readers the auricular points-prescriptions (or combined with body points-prescriptions) most commonly used in acupuncture anesthesia of various kinds of surgical operations are listed as follows:

The Most Commonly used Auricular points- prescriptions (or combined with Bps.-prescriptions) Used in Acupuncture Anesthesia

Kinds of Operation	Eps. Prescription	Bps. Prescription
Exstirpation of tumors of the cerebral hemisphere, exstirpation of tumors of the sella turcica, other intra and extra cranial operations of the frontal and parietal part.	Shenmen* → Kidney; Brain stem (or Forehead; Vertex) → Subcortex; Sympathy, Lung. Compound prescription: Shenmen → Kidney; Forehead → Occiput.	(1) 141 (SI 18); (2) 141 (SI 18); 228 (GB 41); 185 (S 43); 322 (LV 3). (3) 223 (B 2); 195 (GB 8); 121 (SC 21) → 189 (GB 2), 8 (TU 20). 84 (LI 4); 68 (P 6) (all are the normal side).
Operations on the posterior cranial fossa, intra and extra cranial operations of the occipital part	(1) Shenmen → Kidney; Brain stem (or Occiput) → Subcortex; sympathy; Lung. (2) Shenmen, Occiput → Neck; Kidney; Liver. Compound prescription: Shenmen → Kidney; Neck → Occiput.	84 (LI 4); 68 (P 6) (all are the normal side).

* Puncture from a point through to another

	Compound prescription	Points
Cataract extraction	Compound prescription: Shenmen; Lung.	(1) 84 (LI 4); 105 (SC 5); 68 (P 6). (2) 84 (LI 4) (both sides); 223 (B 2) → Yushang; 144 (S 2) (or Chiuhou) → Chienyang. (3) 84 (LI 4); 129 (SI 6) (all are both sides).
Sclera shortening operation	Compound prescription. Eye → Eye 2; Lung (all are at both sides).	84 (LI 4) (both sides).
Iridencleisis		84 (LI 4); 233 (B 2) → Yushang; 149 (S 7); 144 (S 2).
Correction of entropion	Compound prescription: Eye; Eye 1; Eye 2; Liver; Kidney.	84 (LI 4); 68 (P 6); 224 (GB 37); 322 (LV 3).
Curettement of hordeolum	Compound prescription: Shenmen; Lung	84 (LI 4); 106 (SC 6).

Kinds of Operation	Eps. Prescription	Bps. Prescription
Surgical correction of strabismus		84 (LI 4); 106 (SC 6); 201 (GB 14) → Yuyao; 144 (S 2) → 143 (S 1).
Dacryocystorhinostomy		84 (LI 4) (both sides); 233 (B 2); 144 (S 2).
Other operations on the eye	Shenmen; Sympathy (or Lung); Forehead → Eye 1; Eye 2. Compound prescription: (1) Eye (2) Shenmen; Lung.	84 (LI 4); 106 (SC 6); 224 (GB 37). (1) 84 (LI 4) (both sides); Yushang; 232 (B 1). (2) 84 (LI 4); 106 (SC 6).
Tympanotomy		84 (LI 4) (both sides).
Mastoidectomy		84 (LI 4); 68 (P 6); 186 (S 44) (all are both sides).
Rhinotomy, Exstirpation of tumor of the nostril	Compound prescription: Maxilla → Forehead; Adrenal gland → Internal nose; Shenmen → Sympathy.	145 (S 3) → 144 (S 2); 84 (LI 4); 106 (SC 6).

Extraction of rhinopolypus, Correction of septum nasi	(1) External nose → Internal nose, Apex of tragus; Lung, Sympaphy (both sides) (2) External nose → Internal nose; Apex of tragus; Lung; Sympathy.	(1) 84 (LI 4) (both sides); (2) 84 (LI 4); 100 (LI 20); (both sides or affected side). (3) 84 (LI 4); 126 (SI 3) (both sides).
Radical operation of the maxillary sinus	Compound prescription: (1) Adrenal gland → internal nose; Maxilla → Forehead (all are both sides) (2) Maxilla; External nose → Internal nose; Shenmen → Sympathy; Kidney (all are both sides)	145 (S 3) → 144 (S 2); 34 (LI 4); 106 (SC 6). 84 (LI 4); 68 (P 6).
Exstirpation of the maxilla, Radical operation of the maxillary sinus	Compound prescription Maxilla; Kidney (all are affected side); Sympathy → Taiyang.	84 (LI 4); 68 (P 6); 100 (LI 20) (all are both sides or one side) 84 (LI 4); 105 (SC 5); Yatung.

Kinds of Operation	Eps. Prescription	Bps. Prescription
Laryngectomy	Compound prescription: Adrenal gland → Pharynx and Larynx; Neck → Soothing asthma; Shenmen → Sympaphy, Lung, Kidney (all are both sides).	84 (LI 4); 106 (SC 6);
Tonsillectomy	Pharynx and Larynx; Tonsil (all are both sides).	(1) 84 (LI 4) (both sides). (2) 106 (SC 6) (both sides). (3) Pientao (both sides).
Pharyngoscopy and Laryngoscopy		(1) 84 (LI 4) (both sides). (2) 84 (LI 4); 68 (P 6). (all are both sides).
Operations of the parotid gland		182 (S 40); 225 (GB 38); 290 (B 60); 322 (LV 3); 185 (S 43); 230 (GB 43).
Operations on the submaxillary region		182 (S 40); 225 (GB 38); 290 (B 60); 322 (LV 3); 302 (SP 4).

Operations on the mandibula		182 (S 40); 225 (GB 38); 290 (B 60); 322 (LV 3); 302 (SP 4); 84 (LI 4); 68 (P 6).
Operations on the temporo-mandibular articulation		182 (S 40); 225 (GB 38); 290 (B 60); 322 (LV 3); 302 (SP 4) (all are affected sides) 84 (LI 4) (both sides).
Repair of buccolabial defect, Repair of harelip, exstirpation of buccolabial Haemangioma	Compound prescription: Corresponding points of the head and face region	(1) 182 (S 40); 225 (GB 38); 84 (LI 4); (all are both sides or one side). (2) 84 (LI 4); 68 (P 6); 66 (P 4) (all are both sides). 84 (LI 4); 68 (P 6)
Exstirpation of mixed tumor of the palatum, Repair of cleft-palate		84 (LI 4); 68 (P 6); 182 (S 40).
Tooth extraction		(1) 83 (LI 3) → 84 (LI 4); (opposite side of the affected tooth).

Kinds of Operation	Eps. Prescription	Bps. Prescription
Upper incisive tooth Lower incisive tooth Upper caine tooth Lower caine tooth Upper bicuspidate tooth Lower bicuspidate tooth Upper molar tooth Lower molar tooth	Compound prescription: Apex of tragus	2 (TU 26) → 100 (LI 20) 28 (JEN 24); 148 (S 6) 2 (TU 26) → 100 (LI 20); 141 (SI 18). 28 (JEN 24) → 147 (S 5); 148 (S 6) 149 (S 7); 141 (SI 18); 28 (JEN 24); 148 (S 6); 141 (SI 18); 148 (S 6); 28 (JEN 24); 148 (S 6); (2) 84 (LI 4) (both sides). 83 (LI 3) → 84 (LI 4) (both sides).
Exstirpation of adenoma of the thyroid gland. Thyroidectomy, Exstirpation of thyroglossal cyst, Fistulectomy of thyroglossal duct	Shenmen; Lung (or Sub-cortex); Pharynx-Larynx; neck (all are both sides or one side).	(1) 98 (LI 18) (both sides). (2) 84 (LI 4); 68 (P 6) (all are both sides or one side). (3) 84 (LI 4) (both sides); 148 (S 6); 218 (GB 31) (all are affected side or both sides).

Operation	Ear points	Body points
Radical exstirpation of adenocarcinoma of the thyroid and radical dissection of the cervical lymph nodes	Compound prescription: Shenmen; Sympathy; Lung; Neck → Clavicle (all are affected side or both sides).	84 (LI 4); 68 (P 6); (all are both sides or affected side). 84 (LI 4); 68 (P 6) (both sides or one side).
Pneumolobectomy, Pneumectomy, thoracoplasty, pneumectomy combined with thoracoplasty, Exstirpation of tumor of the chestwall	Shenmen; Sympathy; Lung; Pingchuan; Kidney; Thorax.	(1) 84 (LI 4); 68 (P 6). (2) 108 (SC 8) → 66 (P 4). (3) Hsia Yifeng. (4) 105 (SC 5) → 68 (P 6). (5) 94 (LI 14) → 114 (SC 14).
Dilatation of the bicuspid valve	Shenmen; Lung; Thorax; Heart (all are left side).	84 (LI 4); 68 (P 6); 106 (SC 6) (all are both sides or left side).
Pericardectomy		(1) 84 (LI 4); 68 (P 6) (all are left sides). (2) 84 (LI 4); 68 (P 6); (all are both sides). 15 (TU 13); 17 (TU 11).

Kinds of Operation	Eps. Prescription	Bps. Prescription
Operation on the esophagus		(1) 84 (LI 4); 68 (P 6); (all are left side). (2) 84 (LI 4); 105 (SC 5); 94 (LI 14); 117 (SC 17) (all are left side).
Simple mastectomy, Extirpation of tumor of the breast	Shenmen; Sympathy; Internal secretion; Thorax; Lung.	84 (LI 4); 68 (P 6).
Repair of perforation of the stomach; Subtotal gastractomy, Gastroentero anastomosis	Stomach; Shenmen; Sympathy; Lung (all are both sides or left side).	(1) 178 (S 36); 179 (S 37); (all are both sides or left side). (2) 178 (S 36); 117 (SC 17); (all are both sides); Point of the incision (burrying a hao-chen in both sides of the incision).
Cholecystectomy, Exploration of the billary passage drainage of the systic duct	Pancreas; Gallbladder; Adbomen; Shenmen; Lung; Subcortex (all are both sides).	178 (S 36); 304 (SP 6); Tannangtien.

Splenectomy	Compound prescription: Shenmen → Gallbladder; Sympathy, Lung and muscle, Relaxation point (i.e. needling the point between Stomach, Liver, and Spleen → Diaphragm.	84 (LI 4); 68 (P 6).
	Compound prescription: (1) Spleen; Triple Warmer; Lung; Sympathy; Shenmen (all are left side).	178 (S 36); 304 (SP 6); 322 (LV 3) (all are both sides). (1) 302 (SP 4) (both sides). (2) 37 (JEN 15); 332 (LV 13); (left) 66 (P 4); 84 (LI 4); 178 (S 26) (all are both sides).
Enterectomy	Shenmen → Abdomen	178 (S 36); 302 (SP 4) or 322 (LV 3); 84 (LI 4); 68 (P 6); (all are both sides).
Appendectomy	(1) Appendix; Mouth (2) Appendix; Abdomen; Shenmen; Lung.	(1) 178 (S 36) (both sides); 213 (GB 20); (2) Lanwei; Neiche matsui point (i.e. 7 tsun above the medial malleolus).

Kinds of Operation	Eps. Prescription	Bps. Prescription
Repair of inguinal hernia	Patella → Abdomen, Sympaphy. Compound prescription: External genital organs; Small intestine; Sympaphy; Lung.	(1) 178 (S 36) (both sides or affected sides); 215 (GB 28) (2) 249 (B 18); 256 (B 25); 315 (SP 15); 215 (GB 28). 178 (S 36).
Intraperitoneal ligation of the faloppian tubes	Ovarium; Shenmen; Lung; Sympathy; (all are both sides).	(1) 178 (S 36); 325 (LV 6) (all are both sides). (2) 178 (S 36); 213 (GB 26) (all are both sides).
Ceasarean section	Uterus; Abdomen; Shenmen; Sympaphy; Lung; Muscle relaxation point.	178 (S 36); 304 (SP 6); 213 (GB 26); Neiche Matsui point (all are both sides).
Hysterectomia and exstirpation of both adnexa		(1) 26 (TU 2); 24 (TU 4); 213 (GB 26); 264 (B 33); or 263 (B 32). (2) 26 (TU 2); 24 (TU 4); 213 (GB 26); 178 (S 36); 304 (SP 6).

Ovarial cystectomy	Compound prescription: Heart; Kidney;	26 (TU 2); 24 (TU 4); 213 (GB 26); 263 (B 32); 178 (S 36) → Neiche Matsui point. 307 (SP 9) → 221 (GB 34).
Pyelolithotomy, Ureterolithotomy	Kidney; Shenmen; Lung; Sympaphy; Triple Warmer; Spleen or Kidney. Compound prescription:	225 (GB 38); 291 (B 60); 336 (K 3); 185 (S 43); 322 (LV 3); 301 (SP 3); 85 (LI 4); 105 (SC 5); 126 (SI 3); 66 (P 4). Corresponding segmental Peishu point or chiachi point (both sides).
Cystolithotomy, Repair of bladder, Cystotomy, Cystoscopy	Bladder; Abdomen; Shenmen; Lung. Compound prescription: Bladder; Shenmen; Subcortex → Lung.	304 (SP 6) (both sides); 49 (JEN 3); 48 (JEN 4). 178 (S 36); 304 (SP 6).

Kinds of Operation	Eps. Prescription	Bps. Prescription
Evertion of the tunica vaginalis testis		(1) 304 (SP 6); 324 (LV 5) (all are both sides); 214 (GB 27); 215 (GB 28). (2) Tikuan; Fourth lumbar vertebrae.
	Compound prescription: Shenmen → Abdomen.	Chiehkou point
Ligating of hemorrhoid	Compound prescription: Lower segment of the rectum; Lung.	261 (B 30) (both sides).
		280 (B 49) (both sides).
Circumcision		(1) 304 (SP 6); 322 (LV 3) (all are both sides); 49 (JEN 3); 48 (JEN 4). (2) Tikuan; Fourth lumbar vertebra.
	Compound prescription: External genital organs; Shenmen; Sympathy; Lung → Subcortex (all are both sides).	In the penis root (2 electric plates, 2–3 cm wide, are placed around the penis root, electric needling).

Exstirpation of the penis		265 (B 34) (both sides); 50 (JEN 2); 51 (JEN 1); Matsui point (1 cm medially to the tuberosity of the ischium).
Episiotomy		304 (SP 6); 322 (LV 3).
Reduction of fracture of the clavicle	Compound prescription: Clavicle; Shenmen; Subcortex (all are both sides).	68 (P 6); 98 (LI 18) (all are both sides).
Closed reduction of the shoulder joint	Shoulder → Shoulder joint; Shenmen; Sympathy; Kidney. Compound prescription: Shoulder → Shoulder joint; Lung; Kidney; Shenmen → Sympaphy.	84 (LI 4); 57 (L 6).
Repair of the bursa of the Shoulder joint		105 (SC 5); 66 (P 4); 57 (L 6); 84 (LI 4).
Manual reduction of fracture of the humerus, open reduction of old fracture of the humerus.	Shoulder → Elbow; Shenmen; Lung; Sympathy; adrenal gland; Kidney.	

Kinds of Operation	Eps. Prescription	Bps. Prescription
	Compound prescription: Shoulder; Arm; Shenmen; Occiput; Apex of the auricle (all are both sides or one side).	Chiehkou points (i.e. several points in the anterior and posterior regions of the shoulder).
Arthroplasty of the elbow	Compound prescription: Elbow → Shoulder; Shenmen; Spleen → Lung, Kidney.	95 (LI 15); Chienchien → Chienhou; 84 (LI 4); 105 (SC 5).
Rectification of the forearm		91 (LI 11) → 74 (H 3); 56 (L 5); 84 (LI 4); Brachial plexus point (i.e. insert a needle in the axilla where the auxillary artery pulsates, both sides).
Amputation of the forearm	Wrist; Shenmen (all are both sides).	56 (L 5); 73 (H 2); Deltoid muscle (i.e. in the midst of the deltoid muscle); Chienchien → (all are both sides). −84 (LI 4); −103 (SC 3).

Operation	Prescription	Points
Reduction of fractures of ulna and radius, Open reduction and fixation of fractures of ulna and radius	Compound prescription: (1) Elbow → Wrist, Lung, Shenmen. (2) Elbow → Wrist, Lung, Kidney.	91 (LI 11); 105 (SC 5); 61 (L 10); 84 (LI 4); Deltoid muscle; 53 (L 2). 84 (LI 4); Pichung; 91 (LI 11); 95 (LI 15); 113 (SC 13). 68 (P 6) ——105 (SC 5).
Excision of the head of the radius	Elbow; Wrist; Shenmen; Kidney; Subcortex.	
Tendon grafting of the wrist, Division of adhesions		97 (LI 17).
Exstirpation of tumor of the arm	Compound prescription: Lung → Subcortex; Shenmen → Sympathy, Kidney.	186 (S 44); 254 (B 23); 336 (K 3) (all are both sides). 221 (GB 34); 285 (B 54); 178 (S 36).
Exstirpation of tumor of the thigh		178 (S 36); 291 (B 60); Heting.

Kinds of Operation	Eps. Prescription	Bps. Prescription
Ligation of the great saphenous vein	Shenmen → Coxae joint; Abdomen → Knee, Lung, Subcortex.	
Internal nail fixation of intracapsular fracture of the neck of the femur	Buttock → Ankle, Shenmen, Lung, Sympathy, Kidney, Adrenal gland.	(1) 178 (S 36); 182 (B 40); 290 (B 59); 223 (GB 36); 226 (GB 39); 304 (SP 6); 227 (GB 40); 185 (S 43). (2) 221 (GB 34); 182 (B 40); 324 (LV 5); 12th Huato chiachi; 13th Huato chiachi. (3) 221 (GB 34); 226 (GB 39); Hsiafenglung (all are affected side) 325 (LV 6) (normal side).
Amputation of lower part of the thigh	Compound prescription: Knee, Shenmen, Lung. Coxae joint.	217 (GB 30); 280 (B 49); 15th Huato chiachi; 16th Huato chiachi.
Meniscectomy of the knee joint		(1) The 3rd lumbar nerve; Femoral nerve; Chiehkou point (both sides of the incision). (2) The 3rd lumbar nerve; 4th

Operation	Prescription	Points
		lumbar nerve; Ischiadic nerve or 282 (B 51).
Amputatio of the lower portion of the leg.	Compound prescription: Knee → Angle, Shenmen, Lung.	217 (GB 30); 280 (B 49); 16th Huato chiachi; 17th Huato chiachi.
Open reduction and fixation of fractures of the tibia and fibula	Compound prescription: Knee → Ankle, Subcortex.	322 (LV 3); 307 (SP 9); 308 (SP 10); 284 (B 53); 217 (GB 30); 173 (S 31).
Fusion of the talocalcaneonavicular joint	Knee, Ankle, Lung, Kidney. Compound prescription: Toes; Subcortex (all are both sides).	285 (B 54); 288 (B 57); 178 (S 36); 186 (S 44). 321 (LV 2); 230 (GB 43); 304 (SP 6).
Exstirpation of the metatarsus	Compound prescription: Toes (both sides).	(1) 304 (SP 6); 225 (GB 38); 301 (SP 3); 322 (LV 3). (2) 322 (LV 3); 336 (K 3); 226 (GB 39). 302 (SP 4); 304 (SP 6); 221 (GB 34); 182 (S 40) (all are both sides).

Kinds of Operation	Eps. Prescription	Bps. Prescription
Lengthening of the achilles tendon		(1) 285. (B 54); 288 (B 57); 178 (S 36); 186 (S 44). (2) 285 (B 54); 282 (B 51); 178 (S 36).
	Compound prescription: Ankle; Shenmen; Occiput; Lung; Sympathy.	183 (S 41); 336 (K 3); 178 (S 36); 304 (SP 6); 179 (S 37) (all are both sides).
Fusion of vertebral column, Decrompression of vertebral disk, Evacuation of tuberculosis of the vertebral column, Exstirpation of lumbar intervertebral disk	Compound prescription: (1) Shenmen → Symppaphy, Thoracic vertebra (or lumbar vertebra) Lung; Kidney. (2) Shenmen → Kidney; Spleen → Lung (all are both sides).	84 (LI 4); 105 (SC 5) (all are both sides); Chiehkou point. 84 (LI 4); 68 (P 5); Tachui pang (i.e. 0.5 cm from the Tachui point); 126 (SI 3) (all are both sides).
Operation on the spinal cord	Vertebral column (take the corresponding points); Shenmen → Kidney; Occiput → Subcortex, Sympathy (or Lung).	

Supplement : Methods of Acupuncture Anesthesia

I Advantages of acupuncture anesthesia

Basing on our extensive clinical experience, we are of the opinion that acupuncture anesthesia has the following advantages:

(1) It is a safe anesthetic method with a wide range of indication. Not a single death due to such anesthesia occurred in the 80,000-old cases operated on in Shanghai district. It is free from accidents causes by overdosage or hypersensitivity to drugs. Since there was no disturbance of physiologic functions due to drug inhibition on the activities of the nervous, respiratory and circulatory systems, postoperative complications such as respiratory tract infections, pneumonia, abdominal distension and urinary retention were markedly reduced.

Acupuncture anesthesia is especially suitable for patients who are complicated with hepatic, renal or pulmonary dysfunction, or are aged, debilitated, seriously ill or in shock condition, and for those unfit for drug anesthesia because of hypersensitivity or poor tolerance.

(2) There is less embarassment of physiologic functions, which benefits the patient's recovery. In 100 cases of mitral commissurotomy performed under acupuncture anesthesia, blood pressure remained quite stable. Even during intracardiac manipulations, there was only a transient blood pressure drop, and in most cases it rose spontaneously afterwards. This compares favourably with the more protracted blood pressure drop under general anesthesia when pressor drugs are usually needed. Patients after acupuncture anesthesia can eat and move about early; this assists the recovery process.

(3) Under acupuncture anesthesia neither the central nervous system nor the peripheral nervous system as a whole is inhibited, the patient remains awake and can cooperate with the surgeons. During total laryngectomy, the patient may swallow freely, any leakage of saliva can be discovered in time. Also, during operation for correction of strabismus or for artificial vertebra replacement after resaction of vertebral tumors, timely examinations of eye movements or limb functions can be made to ensure better operative results.

(4) Acupuncture anesthesia does not call for complicated anesthetic apparatuses and is not limited by want of equipment of geographical conditions. It is easy to manage and economical. Besides urban areas, it is suitable for use in the countryside and mountainous regions.

2. Methods of Acupuncture Anesthesia

In China, acupuncture anaesthesia is now extensively used in a great number of medical establishment, for people of all ages, from very young babies to people above eighty. It has been used successfully in head, chest, abdominal surgery and 200 other kinds of major and minor operations, in both mild and serious cases.

The most commonly used methods of acupuncture anaesthesia are as follows:

Preparation before Operation

Prior to operation the patient should be needled one to several times (the "needling test"), in order to find out his tolerance of and adaptability to acupuncture stimulation. At the same time, the operative procedure and the ractions he may have during the operation should be explained to him so as to ease his anxiety and win his cooperation.

Selection of Acupuncture points

At present there are varieties of acupuncture anaesthesia with different ways of selecting acupuncture points.

This article introduces only body acupuncture and ear acupuncture currently employed in China. Points are selected along the meridians on the trunk and extremities in body acupuncture and on the auricula in ear acupuncture. These two methods are sometimes used in combination.

Body acupuncture anaesthesia. The following principles have been generally adopted.

(1) Selection of points along the meridians. This is based on the chinglo theory: "wherever the chinglo traverses, therein lies the amenability of treatment." Acupuncture points are selected along the related meridians. In general, acupuncture points with strong induction and good analgestic effect are selected along the meridians intercepted by or in the vicinity of the incision, and also the meridians related to the Tsangfu (i.e. solid and hollow organs) to be operated on. For instance, in gastrointestinal operations, Tsusanli-178 (S 36) of the stomach meridian is selected. Sometimes points near the site of operation are added to strengthen the effect of local analgesia.

(2) Selection of points by the "piencheng" method. Points are selected according to the "piencheng" method in Chinese traditional medicine, i.e., first distinguish the relationships between the symptoms of disease of the responses of the patient during operation and the Tsangfu and Chinglo, and then determine the involved points according to the principles of Tsangfu functions and their interrelations. This method is usually used in co-ordination with the first concept. Thus in cardiac and pulmonary operations, Hsimen-66 (P 4) of the envelope of the heart meridian is selected.

(3) Selection of points according to the segmental distribution of the spinal nerves. Points are selected in the same or neighbouring segmentally innervated areas. For instance, in thyroid operation Futu-98 (LI 18) is selected.

Ear Acupuncture Anaesthesia

Acupuncuture points on the auricle are distributed schematically. Every part of the body has its representative area on the auricle. The points may also be selected according to the method of Tsangfu, Chinglo and Piencheng.

(1) Auricular points selected according to the site of operation. The site of incision and that of the organ to be operated on have corresponding points on the auricle. Similarly, for certain diseases there are responsive points on the auricle. For instance, Eps Stomach or Abdomen is selected in subtotal gastrectomy.

(2) Auxiliary points. Based on clinical experience, Eps Shenmen and Sympathy are considered to have better analgesic sedative effects on the whole body and are selected frequently as auxiliary points.

Acupuncture Stimulation

Needling, The depth of needling should be determined according to the habitus of the patient and the site of acupuncture, generally between 1 and 3 cm. The insertion should be done swiftly and accurately, followed by rotating to and fro slowly with lifting and thrusting movements to produce a feeling of soreness, distension and heaviness in the patient.

Methods of Stimulation. After a needling sensation is obtained, the patient is subjected to stimulation by hand maneuver (or by mechanical manipulator stimulating hand maneuver) or to electric pulse stimulation.

(1) Hand maneuver. It is the fundamental method of acupuncture stimulation, in general, the needle is held with the thumb, index and middle fingers, and stimulation is performed by lifting, thrusting and rotating movements. An experienced acupuncturist is always able to perceive the decreasing and disappearing of "needling sensation" of the

patient, and adjusts the stimulation in time. The frequence of needling is generally maintained at 100-200 movements per minute, the range of rotation between 90° and 360°, and the depth of lifting and thrusting below 10mm. The hand maneuver should be smooth and even, the shaft and the tip of the needle should be kept in the same direction. The strength and speed of the hand maneuver are adjusted according to the operative procedure and the patient's response, so that he is able to tolerate it.

(2) Electrical pulse stimulation. The inserted needle is connected to an electric pulse stimulator and a pulsatile current is used. The output of the electric acupuncture apparatus currently in use is generally in the form of biphasic spike waves, biphasic square waves of sinusoid waves. The frequency of the electric pulses ranges form dozens per minute to hundreds per second. On application, the intensity is initially adjusted to a minimum, and then increased gradually. Most patients report a feeling of numbness and distension. The intesnity of electrical stimulation is adjusted to such an extent that the local musculature quivers slightly and the patient experiences a moderate degree of irritative sensation. However, this sensation often tends to decrease or disappear, therefore the intensity of electrical stimulation should be adequately increased from time to time, or an intermittent electrical stimulation should be applied.

Intensity of stimulation
As the response to acupuncture stimulus varies greatly in different patients, the intensity of stimulation, manual or electrical, should be governed by the habitus and general condition of the patient, as well as by his sensitivity and tolerance to acupuncture. In addition, the irritative effect of operative trauma to the body and the duration of operation should also be taken into consideration.

Induction. Prior to operation, preliminary stimulation, is performed on the selected points for a certain period of time, in order to render the patient adaptable to further acupuncture stimulations gradually, thus producing a good analgesic effect. The induction time is generally 15-30 minutes.

Adjuvant Drugs

Like other anaesthetic methods, adjuvant drugs such as meperidine may be required for acupuncture anaesthesia before and during operation. Our experience indicates that in patients who develop reactions to operative procedures such as incision or suturing of peritoneum, elevating of periosteum and forceful traction of viscera, local infiltration or nerve blocking with anaesthetics may be employed. Some patients may undergo acupuncture anaesthesia successfully without any adjuvant drug during the entire procedure. (For the detail please refer to the book entitled "The Principles and Practical Use of Acupuncture Anesthesia" published by Medicine and Health Publishing Co., Hong Kong.)

Appendix 2

AURICULOTHERAPY USED

IN CURING ADDICTS

WITH ASTONSHING RESULTS

Supplement: Two points-prescription for the treatment of drug addiction

Three weeks ago a 17-year-old student dying from a heavy heroin overdose was admitted in a coma to the Army General Hospital in Bangkok. Instead of putting him in the intensive care unit, usual practice in an emergency. Dr. Aroon Shaowwnasai, chief hospital psychiatrist, treated him on the sopt with acupuncture. Ten minutes later the boy opened his eyes and he is now well on his way to recovery.

The Bangkok hospital where Dr.Aroon works is one of the first in the world to use acupuncture as a serious treatment for drug addiction. American-trained Dr. Aroon got the idea just over a year ago from a Chinese acupuncturist in Hongkong. Ignoring sceptics on his staff who favoured curing addicts with tranquillisers and methadone, he used it on patients with astonishing results.

He cured virtually every heroin and opium addict with acupuncture within 15 days— the exceptions being young addicts in their teens. Finding either they lacked the necessary confidence in the cure or that they were afraid of the needles, he put them on methadone.

When he uses acupuncture on a patient, Dr. Aroon, 45, inserts a needle in the soft part of each ear and connects it with wire to a regulator. This instrument, not unlike a portable radio in size and appearance, operates off a six-volt torch battery. By turning its dials Dr. Aroon adjusts the strength and frequency of the current until it is to the liking of the patient. He leaves the machine running for about 30 minutes.

Usually, he says, the first withdrawal symptoms, blackouts, difficulty in breathing and goose, pimples, start to disappear three minutes after the ear puncturing. After six minutes abdominal pain is reduced and after 15 minutes the patient is feeling quite well, his dizziness and muscular aches gone. The treatment makes him drowsy.

Dr. Aroon repeats the acupuncture process two or three times a day during the first three days after the patient's admission and once daily thereafter. Its chief drawback as a drug addiction cure is that it is time-consuming and laborious.

Although he does not pretend to know its secret, Dr. Aroon firmly believes acupuncture treatment for drug addiction is whorthy of further study and experimentation. The invention of a larger regulator capable of use by several patients simultaneously, wound be especially useful, he maintains.

—From Ta Kung Pao (English edition), Hong Kong, 1975

Supplement: Two Points-Prescriptions for the Treatment of Drug Addiction

Priscription 1.

Acupuncture treatment for detoxication may be divided into two kinds: body acupuncture treatment and ear acupuncture treatment:

A. Points-Prescription of Body Acupuncture:

Anmien, Tachui-14 (TU 14), Neikuan-68 (P 6), Yangling-chuan-221 (GB 34), Sanyinchiao-304 (SP 6), Hoku-84 (LI 4), Jenchung-2 (TU 26) and Kungsun-302 (SP 4).

The needling method is the same as general acupuncture treatment, for instance, strong stimulation and twist the needle continuously, etc.

B. Points-Prescription of Ear Acupuncture:

Ear-Shenmen, Sympathy, Lung, Heart, Subcortex, Brain and Occiput, etc. Twist the needle continuously or use electro-stimulation with adjustable wave:

The frequency of needling is generally maintained at more than 200 movements per minute. Once lasts 10—40 minutes 2—4 times a day, and then the duration and the number of treatment should be reduced gradually until the drug addict is completely released.

According to a detoxicated case report in 40 cases with acupuncture by the concerning Hospital in Hongkong that the successful rate of detoxication was as high as 100%. Observation had been taken more than a year, among them only 8 cases had received more 1—2 treatments, while the rest had no requirement, the result was excellent.

Priscription 2.

Primary points: Tachui-14 (TU 14); Neikuan-68 (P 6), Hoku-84 (LI 4) and Lienchuan-29 (JEN 23).

Auxiliary points: For restlessness, add Shenmen-78 (H 7); mental confusion, add Anmien 1, 2, Yamen-13 (TU 15); vision obscure, add Chingming-232 (B 1) and Chengchi-143 (S 1); tears much, add Yinghsiang-100 (LI 20) through to Pichuan; abdominal pain and vomiting, add Chungwan-40 (JEN 12) and Shangchu-hsu-179 (S 37); Hypotension, add Suliao-3 (TU 25); cold feeling on the skin, add Feishu-244 (B 13) and Chihai-46 (JEN 6); spasm, add Chihtse-56 (L 5) and Chengshan-288 (B 57).

Procedure: 1-3 times daily, with strong stimulation, after twist the needle continuously 1-2 minutes, retain the needle half an hours then twist it again or combined needling with the pulsating currents. A course can be given consisting of 15 days.

Remarks: Parallel with acupuncture treatment, toxic drug must be brought off to the addict or needling it combined with a proper amount of methadone to releave the symptom in the duration of detoxication. After the symptom disappears, it needs continuously 1-2 courses of treatment to consolidate the therapeutic results. Generally speaking, compared with the opium addict, the heroin addict requires larger amount of stimulation, of which the course is also longer. If it is combined with needling the auricular points of Shenmen, Lung and Sympathy, the result will be certainly better.

Appendix 3

INTRADERMAL NEEDLE-THERAPY

Intradermal needle therapy is a method of treatment developed from the curing methods of retaining the needle in ancient China.

This therapy is done by placing a specific-made small needle under the skin where the acupuncture points situated for a rather long time, so it is also called the "Imbedding needle" therapy.

In clinical practice, the symptoms, which need the needles to be retained in the superficial layer of the skin for a long period, are commonly treated with this curing method that is also generally used in auriculotherapy.

(I) Needles and Applications

The intradermal needles have two kinds namely the grain shape needle and the press needle. When not being used, the needles may be immersed in 70% alcohol to be sterilized for future use. (See Fig. 1)

1. Grain shape needle

During treatment, the needle is clipped with a forceps and inserted transversely along the intraderma. It may be imbedded about 0.8-1.3 cm. deep and fixed it up with an oblong adhesive plaster along the direction of the needle.

2. Press needle

This is suitable for superficial insertion in a vertical direction. During treatment, the needle-ring is clipped with a forceps or with fingers, place the needle-tip accurately into the selected acupuncture point. After a light twisting, press the needle up and fix it tightly with an oblong adhesive plaster, finally fix the plaster on a selected acupuncture point. It is important that the region of points selected should not interfered with the normal movements of the limbs. Generally, the points on the back, limbs and ears are mostly adopted.

The duration of imbedded needles may be determined in accordance with the condition of disease. Commonly, 1-3 days, at most 6-7 days. In the hot season, it is not allowed to be too long to avoid infection.

Imbedding the intradermal needle may also be linked with the source of electric current. The strength of the current should be adjusted to the required amount. Duration of treatment is generally from 15 to 20 minutes.

(II) Indications

In clinical practice, this curing method is suitable for the treatment of some painful diseases which are necessary to imbed the needle for a long time, such as neurotic headache, migraine, stomachalgia, biliary colic and also indicated for chronic diseases, such as neurasthenia, hypertension, asthma and irregular menstruation, etc.

(III) Precautions

1. Once 1-2 points, generally it is done on single side or either sides in alternation.

2. Before imbedding the needle, select the region where the needle may be fixed easily and at the same time will not to impede the movements of the limbs.

3. After the needles having been imbedded, if the patient has a feeling of tingling pain or the needle interfere with the movements of the limbs, the needles must then be withdrawn and to be imbbed again.

4. Before treatment, the needle-body should be examined thoroughly to prevent the accident of breaking of the needle.

[SUPPLEMENT]

Method of intradermal imbedding of needle: For this method a fine needle (hao chen) No. 30-32, which is tenecious and uneasy to be broken, is used to be inserted into the selected point. After menipulation, lifting it to the intraderma then along the skin it is inserted again horizontally about 5 fen deep. Finally fix it up with a piece of adhesive plaster, so as not to drop it away. Generally the needle may be retained there for 1-3 days.

Appendix 4-A

MY EXPERIENCE WITH ACUPUNCTURE

Letter from Peking
By Julan Schuman

Having got rid of a shoulder ache after some needles were stuck into me a few years ago. I recently took my bi tze bu tung (clogged nose) in for acupuncture treatment.

The needle

Acupuncture is the ancient Chinese method of inserting and manipulating thin needles, some long, some shorter, into specific body points to cure a string of ailments and some diseases—among them dizziness, headaches, some forms of deafness and paralysis as well as problems of the respiratory system and visual organs.

Books referring to acupuncture were being read in the Sung dynasty (960-1280). The theory is that the human body is an organic unity and sickness can be brought on by imbalance in the body. Stimulating the higher nervous system affects the general physiology and can help restore balance by removing the causes of congestion or antagonism.

No pain

My previous encounter with the slim needle after heat treatment failed had turned out successfully and with virtually no pain. The needling took about 20 minutes every other day for a week. A sterilized, stainless steel needle was used, inserted one time at the point of my ache, another time above and then below it. There was a slight pain as the more than 2-inch needle entered and then a tingling for about a minute in the area of my ailment. Nothing was felt after that.

Though there was some improvement when the session was over, the ache had not completely disappeared. After a while the shoulder bothered me less and less. In a few weeks it was as good as new.

All this does not mean acupuncture always works or it never hurts. Acupuncture for the same problem can be effective for some and not for others. As to pain, it all depends on what is being treated and where the needle are inserted. In general most of the pain comes when the needle first enters.

Dr. Shieh

Needling for my blocked nasal passage was recommended by Dr Shieh—he had worked on my shoulder— after nose drops proved ineffective. Trained in Western medicine in China, he has been practicing acupuncture as well as general medicine for over 16 years.

The clinic he works in is less than a 10-minute walk from my residence and treats Chinese and foreigners. When I walked into the doctor's room, a man was sitting with two or three needles protruding from his skull.

For me, two short needles were inserted, one below each nostril. Whatever my threshold of pain, it was immediately reached as one then the other needle went in, each twirled for a few seconds. Though it didn't lift me out of my chair, it hurt. According to the doctor, the early seconds are when the eyes should tear.

Following the opening of proceedings, there was scarcely anything felt while the needles remained in my face for 15 minutes. The course called for coming in five times, every other day. While my nose was not completely cured at the end, there was decided improvement, at least to the extent of not keeping me awake at nights.

Vital Inserting points

Though I haven't had any personal experience with it, acupuncture is used for treating ailments like bronchitis and insomnia. For those plagued by sinusitis, needles are inserted over a one to two week period on both sides of the nose, into the centre of the skull and between the thumb and forefinger of each hand. This last section, the Hoku (valley between), is a favourite needle target. Pressing down in this area, I've been assured, cures dizziness.

Another vital point is the Neiting (inner household or inner palace). Victims of headaches, stomachaches, toothaches, dysentery and tonsilitis get the needle at the Neiting which is less than an inch above the centre between the second and third toes of each foot.

Whatever the success of acupuncture for various ailments and diseases, it is only in the last few years that needling has been widely and successfully used as a means of anaesthesia in surgery.

Foreign visitors amazed

Ever since 1971 foreign visitors have been amazed and impressed, doctors included, as they filed into operating rooms to watch. Heart, brain and chest operations, appendectomies, and the removal of cataracts, ovarian cysts, thyroid tumors and gallbladders in which no drugs were used all have been seen.

Witnesses to such surgery have told me that quite often patients, wide-awake while being cut open, talk with doctors. In a number of cases, they got up from the operating table, shook hands with the visitors and then walked off, a bit wobbly, to their wards.

Acupunctural anaesthesis instead of drugs has become

more common. However, it is admitted that it can not be used on some patients, and that all is not perfection. At times some pain is felt. Someone who underwent minor surgery with acupuncture told me the cold knife could be felt when it touched the area being operated one.

A few years ago analgesia was induced only by inserting needles into the body and ears. This has been extended to the face and nose. The needling is done either manually or by electricity.

Break through during Cultural Revolution

Acupuncture began to get more attention in 1958 when emphasis was placed on doctors trained in Western medicine studying Chinese medicine. But it was not until the early years of the Cultural Revolution in the late 1960s and the compaign for a big expansion of medical personnel in the rural areas that the real breakthrough took place.

The tremendous spurt in the use of acupuncture was a by-product of the nationwide compaign to build up a medical service in the vast hinterland, where four out of five Chinese live.

Apart from not leaving drug after-effects, acupuncuture anaesthesia is safe, effective, easy to administer and eco-nomical-all of which make it highly suitable for China's rural areas. Every one of the country's well over a million barefoot doctors (paramedical personnel) is versed in the art of needling.

Practised by dentists

Though far from perfected, something new has been added in recent years. Use of acupuncture by dentists has been under investigation. Needles at certain points on either jaw, it is claimed, can produce sufficient numbness of the mouth while teeth are being worked on.

Acquaintances who have seen it done tell me that pressure

applied to needling points can bring on numbness long enough to pull a tooth. However, they hasten to add, it is pretty much in the experimental stage.

Acupuncture for dentistry, at least for foreigners, still is not widely used. Should the experiments bear fruit, those of us who dread the though of having a tooth yanked may some day be able to sit in the dentist's chair far more easily.

Earlier this year when I had to have a tooth nerve removed, the dentist gave me a shot of novacaine. He did not suggest acupuncture or pressure. Until the investigations and experiments get further along, I wasn't going to insist.

—*From Ta Kong Pao (English edition), Hong Kong, 1975*

Appendix 4-B

BRITISH ACUPUNCTRISTS

ON CHINESE ACUPUNCTURE

China has made some new development in her use of acupuncture and her scientists are devoting themselves to a comprehensive theoretical study on this traditional Chinese medical art. Joseph Goodman and William Wright, two members of a British acupuncture delegation said to our reporter when they arrived recently in Hongkong after a threeweek tour of China.

Both Joseph Goodman and William Wright are British acupuncturists and osteopaths. All members of the delegation have in fact engaged in related studies and researches for eight to twelve years. Some of them teach acupuncture in schools in Britain. While touring China, they visited Peking, Shanghai, Tientsin and Kwangchow where they exchanged experiences and skills with Chinese medical workers.

Joseph Goodman and William Wright agreed that, with the encouragement and promotion of the Chinese Government, traditional medical science and traditional Chinese medicine, acupuncture in particular, have advanced by leaps and bounds.

They discovered in China two new features in the skill of acupuncture, One is that acupuncturists there begun to use needles as long as 12 inches to treat certain ailments. With these long needles, the patients can be given more stimulation and the cure may be better effected. Secondly, Chinese acupuncturists treat ailments in certain parts of the body by inserting needles into specific points in the head. They said over 30 points on the top of a person's head have been located. Using needles to stimulate these points can cure not only ailments in the head, but also those in the respiratory system, auditory organs and visual organs.

The two British acupuncturists emphasized that by integrating Chinese medicine with Western medical skill, good effects can be obtained, such as in the treatment of appendicitis and stomach ulcer.

Joseph Goodman pointed out: Besides all this, Chinese are making every effort in research to formulate a comprehensive theory for acupuncture. If they succeed, it would be a great contribution to the medical science, he said.

—From Ta Kung Pao (English edition), Hong Kong, 1975